Most people have no idea what's involved with caring for a loved one with Alzheimer's, that is--until it affects them personally. In this powerful and educational book, Betty describes with stark honesty how caregivers often have to examine life-long values and ideas--just to survive. It's about courage, grit, coping, and how life's unforeseen difficulties force us to change gears with our best-laid plans. Betty writes about her husband, I wrote about my parents, but the theme is the same--that of undying love that even the ravages of dementia are unable to diminish.

—Jacqueline Marcell, author, *Elder Rage*, and host, *Coping With Caregiving* Internet Radio Program

ALZHEIMER'S SURGERY

AN INTIMATE PORTRAIT

AN INTIMATE PORTRAIT OF A PERFECTLY NORMAL, INTELLIGENT, HEALTHY, PHYSICALLY AND MENTALLY ACTIVE MAN AFFLICTED WITH ALZHEIMER'S DISEASE, AND HOW IT AFFECTED HIM AND THOSE WHO LOVED HIM

BETTY WEISS

1663 Liberty Drive, Suite 200
Bloomington, Indiana 47403
(800) 839-8640
www.AuthorHouse.com

AuthorHouse™
1663 Liberty Drive, Suite 200
Bloomington, IN 47403
www.authorhouse.com
Phone: 1-800-839-8640

AuthorHouse™ UK Ltd.
500 Avebury Boulevard
Central Milton Keynes, MK9 2BE
www.authorhouse.co.uk
Phone: 08001974150

ISBN: 1-4208-5795-9 (sc)

First published by AuthorHouse 2/13/2006

Library of Congress Control Number: 2005905086

Printed in the United States of America
Bloomington, Indiana

This book is printed on acid-free paper.

Also by Betty Weiss

When The Doctor Says, "Alzheimer's"
Your Caregiver's Guide to Alzheimer's & Dementia

Front Cover Photos: In grade school, the children teased me, "Bernie Weiss loves you, ha, ha, ha, ha, ha." One christmas, he rode his bike to my house and gave me a brooch encrusted with red stones; I still see it in my mind's eye, but I never wore it and don't remember whatever happened to it. I had no feelings about it. I was too interested in seeing how high I could climb a tree or how long I could hang upside down by my knees on the monkey bar. But by the time we graduated high school, I knew I'd spend my life with him. In middle-age, our family life was ordinary and uneventful. The last photo was taken shortly after he was diagnosed with 'short-term memory loss.' Everyone said there was nothing wrong with him. Often it seemed that way to me, too. Most of the time he was perfectly normal--or so I thought. bw

MATT

You don't raise heroes, you raise sons.
And if you treat them like sons,
they'll turn out to be heroes,
even if it's just in your own eyes.

Walter Schirra, Sr.

WHEN YOU LEAVE ME

Will it be spring, when all the world is green again,
the fragrance of lilacs and roses fills the air?

Or summer, when the air is rich and warm
with gardens and orchards abundant everywhere?

Or autumn, when the gold and red of trees shine
through early morning frost, the fog and rain?

Or the cold, snowy winter when life stands still, hi-
bernates, and waits for spring?

Would I want the sun to shine, the streams to flow,
the birds to sing, or will I hate them for remaining

When you leave me?

Maybe I would rather see the storm, with the rain
pouring out my grief

When you leave me.

But the rain can't stay forever, and the sun will
come again, bringing all the glories,
that will never be the same

When you leave me.

Printed with the permission of the author Eveline Pheanis, caregiver to her Beloved Red.

AUTHOR'S NOTES

My husband had been saying and doing vaguely strange things for a long time before I finally took him to the doctor in 1993. He was diagnosed with 'short-term memory loss.' I was told that there was very little to be done about it, although I tried.

Today's popular Alzheimer's medications were not yet on the market and the reader familiar with the drugs and the disease may wonder why I did or did not do certain things, but I did what I thought was best at the time. Now, a lot more is known, more guidance and information is available, and if I knew then what I learned over the past decade, I may have done some things differently, although I don't know exactly what, it would have still turned out the same.

The reader unfamiliar with Alzheimer's may think that an amazing number of things happened to us, but the truth is I've only written highlights of some events. There was so much more--much, much more--dozens of people who passed through our lives--often close relationships immediately formed and then just as quickly dissolved, although some of them, years later are still intact. There were additional doctors, nurses, coordinators, administrators, therapists, cyberspace friends, counselors, pharmacists, drivers, receptionists, disappearing friends, reporters--print and television--actors, siblings, producers, other caregivers, strangers, professional and non-professional home aides, daycare staffs--professional and volunteer, other Alzheimer's patients, attorneys, relatives who didn't understand and those who tried, accountants, well-meaning people and those who remain indifferent, but if I included everything and everyone in the book, it would make *War and Peace* look like a thank-you note.

Society then, as now, didn't want to hear about Alzheimer's, people didn't believe what I told them, thought a little forgetfulness could be helped with mental stimulation, supplements; and how bad could it be anyway, it's not like there's any disfigurement or physical pain? In the beginning, I thought the same thing.

Fifty years ago, most people could not bring themselves to say the word 'cancer' aloud, it was always whispered, but it didn't stop anyone from getting it, just made care and diagnosis more difficult because of the fear and shame. But now it is spoken about openly, more and more people live longer with cancer, great strides have been made.

So eventually it will be with Alzheimer's. It won't go away if society turns its back in fear and shame. Nearly 1,000 Americans are diagnosed with it every day and with the exception of ongoing research and new medications that will help some people sometimes, most families will continue to trod the same unrelenting path my husband and I took--at least for the foreseeable future.

This book will help people to understand all the impossible things that occur, realize that most of the bizarre happenings are the normal consequence of the disease. It explains the reality of Alzheimer's from an insider's personal experience, a layman's point of view. It will help not only those who have to deal with it, but even more so for those who think either, 'it's no big deal, a little forgetfulness' or 'I'm going to run and hide.'

It's too much for most people and many friends and family simply disappear because they are creeps and you can't give them a 'compassion' transplant; others say, truthfully, that they can't bear to see someone they know and love in such a terrible, dreadful condition--as if it's easy for the caregiver who has to 'see' it all 24/7!

It's simple fear that makes people leave, and to them I say, 'feel the fear but help and visit anyway!' Alzheimer's is not catching. It is one thing to have sympathy for people with a brain disease, but it is quite another thing to shun them, to turn away so that you don't have to look at their mental and physical deterioration. They didn't start out that way, they were perfectly normal people, just like you, and they're still inside; they still need friends, love and attention, maybe more than ever. They did nothing to bring it on, none of it could have been avoided and no one is at fault. If someone you know is dealing with it, it can be depressing, but lots of things are depressing, you don't have to dwell on that. Nor is it the worst thing in the world, although it is certainly up there in the top two or three. I don't mean to minimize it, it's an unvarnished tragedy, but it's also life, part of the good and part of the bad.

The outsider doesn't understand how incredibly difficult it is for the family caregiver, that you have to be on alert 24/7 because something needs your attention *every* minute of *every* day. Professional caregivers have their work schedules and specific duties defined and work with other staff. They get days off, vacations, benefits. It would be against all labor laws for a professional to always be on duty and have to do everything alone the way family caregivers do. Hopefully, this book will open the minds of those who don't believe the caregivers, who don't see the trauma and think it's being exaggerated; everything appears to be going along so well--what's the problem?

Not every Alzheimer's family has gone through what we have; many have gone through much, much worse. And not every caregiver is blessed to have the emotional, physical and emergency support that I had on occasion, nor the financial resources that I was able to muster, although, again, many have much more.

It is getting more and more difficult for society to ignore Alzheimer's, and as our boomers age, the number of its victims will skyrocket, so it is vitally important for *everyone* in society to understand the facts about this illness, whether or not they are personally touched by it.

Alzheimer's hides zealously, is frustratingly vague, gossamer, difficult to see and impossible to define. Hopefully, readers will come away with a sense of its true nature, its secret unknown life so that they will learn how it can happen to a perfectly normal, intelligent, decent, healthy, mentally and physically active man and the impact it had on him and those who knew and loved him.

You can begin reading the story now on Page 1, but the statistics below will help you to understand more.

Betty Weiss

September 2005

STATISTICS

Statistics vary regarding almost everything about Alzheimer's, but the following, gathered from numerous sources not specifically cited, are within the generally accepted norms.

- One out of three Americans knows of someone with Alzheimer's, but the vast majority knows little about the disease and shows scant interest in learning.
- Alzheimer's can begin to attack the brain decades before the first symptoms appear.
- Medicare and almost all medical and hospitalization insurance do not cover the cost of long-term care for most Alzheimer's patients.
- In June 2001, the Alzheimer's Association reported that over 62% of respondents to the question, **"Do you think your physician is knowledgeable about Alzheimer's disease?"** replied **'no.'**
- In 1999, there were 44,536 deaths from Alzheimer's, surpassing the combined total of auto accidents and breast cancer in the United States.
- As of February 2003, in America, Alzheimer's was the fourth leading cause of death, following heart disease, cancer and stroke.
- One in 50 Americans has Alzheimer's. Every day, an average of 986 patients is diagnosed with the disease.
- Three-quarters of home-bound caregivers do not

get consistent help from family members, especially spousal caregivers.

- Estimates are that 5% to 25% of victims have Alzheimer's in the family. To date, there is no known cause for the vast majority of others stricken.
- Depending on where you live, the average annual cost of caring for an Alzheimer's patient is easily $60,000.
- The average length of stay in a care facility is 2 to 3 years but it can often last 6 or 7.
- Today, the annual cost of Alzheimer's care to America is about $100 billion and by mid-century, as the boomers age, the costs are expected to overwhelm the health care system, bankrupting Medicare and Medicaid.
- Forty-three percent of caregivers for Alzheimer's patients fall into a clinical depression that can linger for years, even after the loved one dies.
- Fifteen percent of Alzheimer's caregivers will die before their contemporaries and many will die before the patient they're caring for.
- Elderly caregivers with a chronic illness themselves have a 63% higher mortality rate than their non-caregiving peers.
- The caregiving spouses of Alzheimer's patients suffer from depression at three times the rate of others in their age group.
- In 2002 alone, Alzheimer's cost American business about $61 billion dollars.
- Even if a loved one is cared for in the home, it can easily cost over $100 a day just for an in-home

aide; and medications, supplies, rentals, doctor visits, visiting nurses and more add up to another average of several thousand dollars a month.

- Alzheimer's is the third most expensive disease in the United States after heart disease and cancer.
- Well over 4 million Americans have Alzheimer's.
- 76 million boomers are reaching the age where Alzheimer's is most prevalent. By the time they reach their mid-80's, 50% are expected to have Alzheimer's.
- By 2050, Americans with Alzheimer's are expected to reach 13.2 million.
- Currently there is no cure for Alzheimer's and only a few drugs that can sometimes slow down its progress and maybe reverse, briefly, some symptoms in some patients.
- The current aging population is now more vulnerable to Alzheimer's because drugs and surgeries have been developed to prolong the life of those with cancer and heart disease only to leave them more susceptible to Alzheimer's as they continue to age; along with any residual cancer and heart conditions as well as other diseases like diabetes, and just general aging.
- While it is true that some younger people get Alzheimer's, it is generally considered a disease associated with aging. This trend is likely to continue as more diseases are overcome and more and more people live longer.
- Although 45% of Americans have had personal experience caring for an aging relative, 46% admit they have not planned for the possibility of their

own long-term care. Despite what boomers see happening to their aging parents, they believe it will never happen to them.

- 63% of Americans do not have a will or living trust.
- Most Americans never discuss such issues with their families.
- Caring for a relative with Alzheimer's is so grueling, physically and emotionally, that nearly 75% of caregivers are relieved when their loved one dies.
- Ninety percent of caregivers believed that death was a relief for the patient.
- There are lower rates of depression among those caring for someone with cancer and other terminal diseases than there are for Alzheimer's.
- Those caring for Alzheimer's patients endure the anguish of caring for a loved one who, in many respects, is already gone. To make things worse, the disease often causes patients to seem unappreciative of the enormous sacrifices made for them by the caregiver.
- Half of Alzheimer's caregivers spend 46 hours a week caring for the patient and 59% feel on call 24/7. Alzheimer's caregiving is exceptionally long and demanding.
- In 2003, in the United Kingdom, about 5.9 million people provided informal care for another person. Of those, only 56% were in good health. Conversely, 70% of people giving no care were in good health.
- Again, in the UK, 53,000 boys and 61,000 girls between the ages of 5 and 15 provided informal

care; 18,000 provided 20 hours or more of care a week, 9,000 provided at least 50 hours. The health of 773 of these children under 16 was rated "not good."

- 498,000 men and 539,000 women over 65 were informal caregivers in the UK. Over 1/3 provided more than 50 hours a week, and more than 1/4 rated their own health as "not good."
- Over half of the oldest informal caregivers in the UK, those over 85, provided care of more than 50 hours a week. The health of 1/3 was rated "not good."
- The above informal caregivers, as opposed to paid employees, are in contravention of the European Working Time Directive.
- Alzheimer's is all but a step-child in medical care and research. Far less money and effort are spent on trying to find a cure for it than on other more 'popular' diseases. This mind-set has to change, otherwise, with more and more diseases being cured, with more and more people living longer, with 50% of them destined to suffer and die from Alzheimer's, and substantial numbers of informal caregivers ruining their own health in their caregiving efforts, then what's the point?

"Love is patient, love is kind. It is not jealous or boastful, it is not arrogant or rude. Love does not insist on its own way. It is not irritable or resentful. Love does not rejoice at wrong, but rejoices in the right. Love bears all things, believes all things, hopes all things, endures all things. Love never ends.

1st Corinthians 13

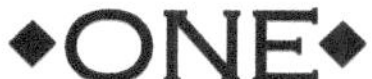

June 1993

Paris, France

Every year we went to Paris. Our daughter Debby lived there and Bernie was familiar with the neighborhood around her apartment. He'd buy *croissants* at the *boulangerie* across the street, walk to *Gare de Lyon* for the English newspaper, pick up the *petits garcons* from the nearby grade school, and discuss computer maps with her husband, Jean-François. We'd walk along the Seine, or watch the mower cut the grass on the sides of the *Palais Omnisports*. But on this trip, our first since his retirement, his behavior was bizarre.

Although it was a straight shot from our hotel to Debby's, Bernie would get confused walking there, once he walked off with a knot of people going in another direction. He'd repeat something immediately after he'd said it, or repeat what someone else had just said, and he wasn't following conversations. Often he seemed apart from whatever was going on and sometimes he talked endlessly.

I asked Debby if she had noticed anything different about her Dad recently, and she said she'd seen odd things for over a year. On the phone, back home in Los Angeles, our son Matt said that he and his pit crew had been re-checking everything Bernie did on our race cars for a long time. So it wasn't just me.

It was easy to attribute his actions to the stress he had about the declining aerospace economy in Southern California and wanting to sell his transformer business during such troubled times. I knew I'd been denying what I saw happening, but sometimes that's just my way. Denial can be a perfectly good defense, and often as not, if I denied something long enough, it went away. But this had been gnawing, it wasn't going away and it couldn't be denied any longer.

Now, whatever 'it' was, it was definitely in my face. I had to find some answers, get my feet on the ground, and I could hardly wait to go home to see our family doctor. I thought I'd started on the road to putting our lives back on track. Instead, I had no idea that I would be embarking on an uncharted journey, the length and depth of which I could never have imagined.

August 1993

Los Angeles, California

The Diagnosis

Once home I wondered if I really needed to call the doctor. Some of the things Bernie did could so easily be explained. Don't we all misspeak, get distracted, turn the wrong way? But I couldn't rationalize away everything that Debby and Matt had said, the strange behaviors, the safety issues at the racetrack.

Dr. Franklin was an old-fashioned family practitioner we'd been seeing for years. He never overprescribed, ordered unnecessary tests or seemed to overreact. On the phone, I told him what had happened in France and that Bernie seemed fine now, he just got confused when we were in a strange place. I could be making a mountain out of a molehill. It wouldn't be the first time.

But the doctor said to come in, so I made an appointment and told him not to tell me if it was Alzheimer's, make something up if you have to, but don't tell me that. I only knew three things about Alzheimer's: (1) There was nothing to be done for it, (2) people forget who their children are, and (3) it could only be diagnosed at autopsy. And I wasn't ready to deal with any of that.

Whether to placate me or not, the doctor said that he doubted it was Alzheimer's. It could be any one of several things, but no matter the cause, the treatment would be the same. While that seemed odd, it was also strangely reassuring. Someone else was going to be responsible.

Bernie and I had never gone into an exam room with each other, but he didn't say a word when I walked in with him this time. There was a brief physical; heart, lungs, throat, ears, all that stuff, and then, quite casually, some chitchat. Bernie didn't object to anything, just went along. When asked, he knew the answers to obvious questions; where he was, the President, Vice-President, current events. He got a little confused on the day and the month, but that can happen to anyone. Then he was asked to count backwards from 100 by sevens. Not a challenge for him, I knew.

Oh, God! Oh, God! A veil was lifting before my eyes. He went to '93' and then the numbers were all wrong. I was trying to count it myself, to mentally retain the necessary simple math while listening to him, but he was all ajumble. He simply couldn't do it! Then he was asked to repeat and remember three simple things like a car, a tree, and a banana. A little more chatting and then the doctor asked him to repeat the three things he'd told him only moments before. Oh, God! He had no memory of what they were, or that he'd even been told! Oh, God!

Somehow, in such simple fashion, and over thirty years of medical practice, the doctor probed into the mind of this intelligent, healthy, capable man and pin-pointed the source of his unusual actions. It was as astonishing to me as pulling a needle out of a haystack on the very first try.

The diagnosis sounded benign enough: 'short-term memory loss.' So, I thought, he forgets. Big deal. But when the doctor suggested a brain scan, that did it! Those two little words, 'brain scan,' hit me like I'd been poked with a cattle prod. I felt a full body assault from my scalp to the soles of my feet, and I knew instinctively that things would never be the same again.

I never realized until that moment how emotionally attached I was to my husband. Sure, I'd thought more than once that something awful might happen to him, that he'd be killed or terribly wounded in Korea, and horrible thoughts could cross my mind when he was really late coming home. But this was not an imagined possibility, this was real. My body reacted even before I had the thought. If I cared less for him, I wouldn't have felt so vulnerable.

The Brain Scan

Now please don't fault me on any medical terminology, but the way I understood it, the brain scan showed that the blood vessels in the area of the brain that control short-term memory had become constricted. That slowed the blood flow which, in turn, prevented enough oxygen from getting through to keep everything working properly. It made sense to me. An oxygen-deprived brain would have to produce some sort of problem.

Why this happened to Bernie, no one really knew, and the brain scan couldn't tell. Having heard a lot more than I ever wanted to hear about memory loss, I concluded on my own that he probably had one or two little silent strokes, most likely brought on by extreme stress. Some doctors claim that stress won't do that. But it didn't really matter. We had to live with it, whatever the cause.

Dr. Franklin gave him two medications, one made the blood slippery so that it could move easier through his system, and the other kept it circulating more readily so that it didn't stay in his lower extremities. Since then, I've been told that such medications wouldn't help, wouldn't change his condition in any way. I knew they were neither a cure nor a prevention, no one ever claimed they were. But imagination or not, I believed that I saw a difference in his mental functioning when he took them. If he forgot, or more accurately when I forgot to give them to him, he seemed to get goofier again--although I'd begun to realize that he went up and down anyway. I'd checked my drug book, they couldn't hurt, they weren't expensive, and it gave him something to do to make him feel like he was helping his condition. Maybe placebos would have done the same thing, but that was the choice I made.

Although Dr. Franklin said he still didn't think Bernie had Alzheimer's, he gave me a book to read about the disease, saying many of the symptoms overlapped and that I'd see the differences, which I did.

He also had Bernie take an echocardiogram. It showed that he had a heart murmur, probably from a childhood disease. He was only 64, and otherwise in excellent health.

During this time, my blood pressure became erratic, only meds kept it in check. And except for Debby and Matt, I never told anyone else anything about any of it.

"You, Me, And The Kids"

I asked Bernie if there was something special that he cared about, something he had always wanted to do. Now that he was retired, there was nothing stopping us. But he said, "All I care about is you, me, and the kids."

Talk about a man having his priorities straight! Just like that he blew off work, sports, travel, hobbies, money, socializing, classes, volunteering--everything except 'you, me, and the kids.' And since I felt the same way, we would simply continue to live the life we had already built together.

On occasion he talked about starting another business. I'd find notes and drawings that he'd scribbled, but when I looked at them, they made no sense. He puttered in the garage, bought little tools and things, but never again did anything substantial.

The Importance Of "Now"

Some people always need something to do. They have to work, they *have* to be busy, like if they're not busy, they're not important, not really living. They dare not waste time--as if serenity is a waste of time. Why do they think they have to be productive every minute, even if it's no more significant than chasing a ball around? Sit still already!

My goal, then, was to *be* with Bernie, not to play a mean game of tennis, trudge a golf course, rush from one event to another, to work when we didn't have to, or drag our clothes halfway around the world just to take our picture in front of some overexposed landmark.

We'd done enough of that already. In the grand scheme of things, all these activities now seemed like meaningless distractions, because if you're really lucky, sometimes there's nothing special you have to do, you can just be with the ones you love, and that so called 'doing nothing' can be a very rare and precious time.

So I sat down with Debby and Matt, told them that nothing was going to change, we'd continue doing our little errands and watching TV game shows. Bernie still played *Wheel of Fortune* quite well, often better than I did. We'd see an occasional movie, take week-end trips, hang out at the racetrack, eat at the same coffee shops, and go to France to play with our little grandsons, Guillaume and Justin. I was perfectly comfortable with all of this.

Hidden Behaviors

It annoyed me no end when Bernie started asking for safety pins and Velcro. He wanted to secure his pants pockets. I'd give him big pins and he'd fuss with them, in and out of the pockets. Or he'd ask me to do something with the pockets, but I could never do it to his satisfaction. I'd ask 'why' but he didn't seem to have an answer.

He always carried a money clip, and on one trip to France he lost it with $300. I was certain it was pinned someplace in his clothes, hidden in the house, didn't think he really lost it, but it was never found. I didn't know, at the time, that 'money' is a big thing with Alzheimer's patients. They worry about it endlessly, think it's been stolen, hide it away and then forget where.

He was, by nature, a very generous man, never stingy, and yet there was always a 'problem' with money. From the start he'd give me his pay check and almost always with the serious admonition to be careful, he didn't know when we'd get any more. I'd often ask him to take over paying the bills, but he never would. If he had to write a check, his hands would tremble, he'd often make a mistake, have to void it, sometimes I thought he'd break out in a sweat. But at the same time, his head was full of mathematical equations, electrical, mechanical and scientific tables and formulas and he'd write them out, pages and pages of them. He'd also write excellent business letters in longhand, so it wasn't the writing or the arithmetic itself--it was only with money, or so it seemed to me. It was easy enough to chalk it up to the '1929 depression,' but he was really too young to remember much about that.

Anyway, I never figured it out and in those early days, never connected this fixation with money to a disease--who would think such a thing? It was just one more thing he did that might sometimes puzzle me, but I found it easier to let it ride. It was no biggie, none of it seemed all that important, it was just his way. There were clues, hidden and overt, but I didn't put it all together, not for a long, long time. It's only now, looking back, that some things have become clear. At the time, there really was nothing to do, we had a good life and I gave it scant thought.

"I Wish You Could Have Known Him Before"

At some point, everyone who has a family member like Bernie will talk about the way he used to be before memory loss stole him away. It's important, because if you don't know what he was like before, then you can't understand the contrast, the devastation, the loss of everything that makes each of us so unique from each another, like a eulogy for someone who's still alive, it has to be said.

Sometimes, I believe, people looked at Bernie and me and thought that we're such a cute little old couple, childhood sweethearts, a real romantic love story, but that's too saccharine. So here's how we really are.

As a very little girl I saw *Gone With The Wind* and when Scarlett stood tall and vowed she'd never go hungry again, I knew that's the way I was. Her strength and resolve thrilled me. At the same time, like Scarlett, I'm well flawed, but those are my secrets.

Thankfully my world has never been destroyed around me and I've never had to claw my way back up. In fact, I've always led a rather sheltered life; although it is my way to daydream a lot, but like Scarlett, to be a realist and pragmatic. I know that many people, especially men, rarely like women like Scarlett. I've lost track of the number of men over the years who have told me that I was too outspoken, too independent for a girl/woman, and told Bernie *in front of me* that he should control me better! Imagine! But with Bernie, I never had to pretend.

Unlike 'Rhett,' Bernie stayed with his 'Scarlett,' he seemed to love and tolerate me when few other men would. I always knew that he preferred me to be 'Betty Crocker,' to have meals on the table, all that *hausfrau* stuff. But the truth is, I'm a disaster in the kitchen. I've been known to burn Jell-O.

Yet, he never complained, never demanded, never yelled. How could I not love someone like that in return? And unlike 'Scarlett,' I knew a good thing when

I saw one. I wasn't about to trade my 'Rhett' for some wimpy 'Ashley.'

I began to fall in love with Bernie while we were in high school. He courted me in a roadster he'd built by himself, rode a motorcycle, wore a black leather jacket, and combed his hair in a ducktail. He was a lot like 'The Fonz' in *Happy Days,* before there even was a Fonz. I thought he was cool, and he loved me.

It wasn't long before we married, had kids, dogs, horses, cars, good times, hard times, successes, failures--but all in all, a pretty decent life for forty years and then everything changed--and, consciously, I never saw it coming.

Subtle Changes

Now that I knew there was 'something,' day by day I was beginning to see changes, but at the same time, I *didn't* see them. It was so simple to dismiss every strange happening, to be reassured when everything was normal, to believe that it was all OK.

On my birthday he went to our neighborhood florist and bought me flowers. See, I thought, he remembered my birthday, he's perfectly fine. The next day, though, looking at the bouquet, he thought that somebody had sent them to him. I didn't correct him, but I felt myself sinking.

Once he bought me a little girl's plastic handbag for $1.49, the price tag was still on it. He was so proud. I told him that I'd use it a lot, but he soon forgot he ever gave it to me.

The worst time though was Christmas when he suddenly realized that he didn't remember to get me a gift. Tears filled his eyes and he cried. He felt so bad, and it hurt so much to see. I told him that it was

OK, hugged and kissed him, but inside I was crying myself.

Bernie was getting worse all the time--but then for a few days he'd be fine--I never knew what would come next. Maybe my world was disappearing around me after all. Poor Scarlett.

Innate Values And Talents

It would be easy to say that Bernie was rigid and let it go at that. But sometimes what seems rigid is really a standard of values. He was honest--always, always, always honest--rigidly honest. He was faithful--always, always, always, faithful--rigidly faithful. He was loyal--always, always, always loyal--rigidly loyal. And he never understood people who were otherwise.

Bernie spent his childhood taking apart radios, watches, and whatever other little things he could find and then putting them back together. As a teen-ager, he could overhaul any Chrysler or GM automobile engine blindfolded.

Eventually he started his own business in our garage, literally with a bag of nuts and bolts he'd bought at a surplus store. Success didn't happen overnight. There were far too many false starts, profound disappointments, never enough money, and countless nights without sleep for both of us. But with his working 16- and 17-hour days and my working as an executive secretary, things finally began to pay off. During those years, I said that I went to bed every night with Johnny Carson, and when Bernie came home at one or two in the morning, I'd be asleep on the couch with the TV on. Then we'd go into the children's room, kiss them each, straighten their covers, and go to bed.

Such a life is not for everyone, I know dull when I see it. But Bernie and I were like a pair of worn slippers nestled together in the back of the closet floor. It's not terribly exciting, but it suited us.

"Okay, Houston, We've Had A Problem Here"

Jack Swigert
'Apollo 13' – 1970
NASA's Official Transcript

When Bernie finally sold his business, he brought home boxes and boxes of mementos. I wish there was a museum for the sort of things he and countless other small subcontractors did in supplying the large aerospace companies. They, unknown and largely unsung, were the people who put the aerospace program on the map--or more accurately--into space.

When Neil Armstrong said, "One giant leap for mankind," it was heard through a communications system with a transformer in it that Bernie designed and manufactured and remains on the moon to this day. Every time Armstrong's voice is replayed, Bernie's contribution is replayed. The words, "Houston, we've had a problem," also came through one of his units. His innate abilities have touched the world. He was part of all that history, his brain was part of it, and when you heard those words and waited breathlessly for the astronauts to return safely from the back of the moon, you were connected to him.

But, eventually his brain became so out of kilter that he couldn't even find the stupid salt shaker where it'd been for over forty years on the stupid kitchen counter.

•TWO•

February 1994

Just What Is Short-Term Memory Loss?

I had absolutely no idea what I was dealing with, so I sent away to medical institutions and universities for White Papers on memory. You think I understood any of it!! Not much after the titles!! I bought transcripts of TV programs about memory and scoured the Internet looking for anything that might help. I visited countless health and government web sites, pulled up articles from medical journals, newspapers, magazines, universities, hospitals--whatever I could find and wherever I could find it. I learned a little more about memory loss, but mostly I learned that there wasn't much anyone could do, especially when you can't pinpoint the cause.

What most people don't understand about short-term memory loss, is the word LOSS. On occasion, we all forget things. Why did I walk into the bedroom? How could I forget to buy bread when that's why I went to the market? Where are my car keys, my eyeglasses, my book? I forget names and birthdays, even my own. I forget words all the time. Sometimes my conversations come to a complete halt while I search my mental memory bank for a word I've used thousands of times but now suddenly eludes me.

This is *not* what was going on with Bernie. Once most people are reminded of something that they forgot, they'll still remember it. Retrace your steps and you'll remember why you went to the bedroom. Put away the groceries and you'll remember you forgot the bread. But with memory LOSS, reminders don't help because the memory has been LOST. It simply doesn't exist, and if it doesn't exist, it can't be retrieved.

As hard as it is living with someone like that, think of the horror it must be for the person who has it. I couldn't even begin to imagine what went on in Bernie's mind, and I didn't want to know. I couldn't bear to think about it. I couldn't deny it, I couldn't control it, but I could accept it--most of the time.

For us, our blessing was that Bernie only had SHORT-TERM memory loss. We went to grammar school together, we'd been together, dating and married, nearly fifty years, if he lost his long-term memory, I'd really be adrift alone. Oh, sometimes he'd forget something in our early years, but mostly he remembered the schools, teachers, friends, family, events. He remembered our cars, of course, places we'd been, and when he was in the Army. So we still had all of that.

It was possible his condition could turn into Alzheimer's, but then that could happen to anyone. He still didn't seem to have most of the classic symptoms. But sometimes it seemed that Bernie forgot he was eating a meal, and if we were at home, he'd just get up from the table and start doing something else. Other times, he'd sit with a forkful of food held in front of him for a long, long time. He'd forget to continue raising the fork all the way to his mouth--right in the middle of the motion--he'd forget what he was doing and just sit.

Or he'd take off a T-shirt, meaning to put on a clean one, but then he'd immediately forget and put the same shirt back on, as if it were the fresh one. He'd put out a clean towel to take a shower, then get dressed instead. Most of the time, though, he did complete his meals, put on clean clothes and shower. He also stopped turning on the TV. I'd turn it on for him, but he'd just sit and sit in front of it, no matter what came on the screen.

Another problem was that I never knew from moment to moment whether he was going to forget something simple or remember something complex. There didn't seem to be any consistency to the behavior of short-term memory loss. He'd remember, he'd forget, he'd remember, he'd forget. I felt like I was trapped inside a giant kaleidoscope being turned by an unseen hand. I recognized the colors, but the patterns wouldn't hold steady. I could see Bernie, but I never knew what he'd be like, he could change on the twist of a wrist.

Getting Understanding

I'm not sure when or exactly why I stopped using the term 'short-term memory loss.' I just got so tired of explaining what it meant. Somewhere from the back of my mind I picked out the word 'dementia' and began using that. It seemed so much easier, so much more definitive, a word that would be taken more seriously, although a surprising number of people had no idea what it meant.

For a long time I couldn't talk to anyone about it, anyway, except for Debby and Matt. No one seemed to notice, and you don't just bring it into a conversation--'oh, by the way, Bernie has short-term memory loss--please pass the peas.'

Eventually, I did try to tell people some of the things that were happening, but they'd stop me with a story about something silly that they themselves did or forgot. Part of it was dismissal and denial, but a lot of it was just not seeing, not understanding. They wanted to tell me their views without really listening to what I had to say.

For the most part, you'll only get understanding from someone who has already walked in the same moccasins. I've always felt that understanding was a funny thing anyway, not really understood, if you will. When we know of starving people, we give our donations and think we understand. Maybe we've missed two or three meals on any given day, so we've known hunger--no doubt about that. But starvation, the end result of hunger--no, I couldn't understand how someone felt because as hungry as I've ever been, I've always known that I'd have something to eat soon enough. I simply couldn't understand what it must be like to be hungry, to know that there would be no food forthcoming, ever.

Often, when I tried to tell people something, they said, and they meant it, that they understood. They understood it for the moment. Maybe they'd nursed someone for a month or two while they regained strength after surgery and knew how difficult that was, or were even caring for someone permanently bedridden who still had all their mental capacity. But they couldn't imagine what it was like to be a caregiver to someone mobile, demented, and getting worse.

I'd ask people not to leave phone messages with Bernie, but they'd say he sounded fine on the phone and they'd leave messages anyway, which I either never got, or were so garbled I couldn't make them out. He couldn't read, follow instructions or dialogue, but people gave him things to read, asked him to do things, invited us to events he couldn't comprehend. They made suggestions--I knew well meaning--but it was all impossible. Bernie looked and acted so normal that I believe they thought they were helping, doing things to keep him busy and stimulated. They couldn't believe that he was unable to *do* anything. Goodness knows it took me long enough to figure it out, and I was living with it day after day.

None of this should be taken as license to stop interacting with people who have dementia. Gifts and social activities can be very important and much appreciated. But if I sound angry, at times I really was. And I admit that much of it was misdirected. I'd like to have been able to hide that part of caregiving--the anger, the frustration--but I don't think I was unusual, and I'll wager that most caregivers feel the same way and are frequently justified.

Dementia, like Bernie's, was not easy to live with, and we know that it lasts as long as the patient lives. Whether or not the caregiver lasts that long is problematic.

A Prisoner In His Own Mind

One of the first things I was told about short-term memory loss was that people who have it keep forgetting that they have it, but I don't believe that's always true. I think Bernie always knew something was happening to his mind, that he was losing control. And while it may be somewhat of a blessing for victims who forget, it's not for the rest of us. We are left to watch helplessly, day by day, hour by hour, as the brain goes into meltdown and steals away the very core of the one you share your life with.

Bernie was so often frightened, terrified, a prisoner in his own mind--I could hardly bear to watch--how could he stand it? And to compound it all, no one noticed. If I'd been on the outside, I suppose I wouldn't have seen it either. What was a little forgetfulness?

If Hollywood made a movie about Bernie's dementia, all you'd see was a character on screen who looked perfectly normal, who spoke in a normal fashion, who appeared to do all the right things. But it'd be an image, no more real than Batman's saving Gotham, because in reality Bernie couldn't do anything right, and his knowing that increased his fear. There was never going to be a feel-good ending, not ever.

"You come home.
The dog throws itself at you.
Where have you been?
You've been gone so long.
I missed you, missed you, missed you.
I love you, love you, love you.
What's in the bag? Something for me?
Oh, let me lick your ear.
Oh, let me chew your gloves.
You're home!"

Pam Brown

We needed a dog, and I wanted a dog-dog, not a little fluff I could put in my handbag, but a dog that took up half the couch and was always underfoot.

I thought it would give Bernie a focus, something to care for, to get outside of himself. And because we've always had dogs, it wouldn't be a new experience, which is really difficult for anyone with dementia.

We went to a doggie orphanage and chose, 'Sophie,' the biggest one they had. She had her bed at the foot of ours, on Bernie's side, and that's where she slept. She was completely loving and devoted.

When another dog came by, she'd bark and tear through the house to the back yard like a runaway locomotive. I'd say, "Go, go, go 'Sophie,' go get 'em." Bernie said, "Be quiet, slow down." When you're a dog you can hear those conflicting messages and it won't mess up your head. Bernie was afraid, with her speed and lack of caution, that she'd hurt herself going through the doggie door or sail through the front window. I didn't think so.

'Sophie' weighed at least 85 pounds, mostly because Bernie forgot when he fed her, so he'd feed her again. They both got so much pleasure from their frequent jaunts to her cookie jar that I was happy to let it be. Usually he'd fix her breakfast in the morning, but on occasion I had to remind him. He never forgot, though, to clean up the yard after she decorated it for him, and that was good. They'd go for walks around the block together. I knew she'd bring him back home, but I had to watch everything. When they came back, he sometimes forgot to take off her leash and it was dangerous to have her roaming around with it.

Bernie, 'Sophie,' and I were a little like *The Three Musketeers*. We did things together, went places together and cared deeply about each other. I realized it wasn't good for her health to be so heavy, but that's the price paid for Bernie's forgetting that he'd fed her. She thought dementia was a swell thing.

Taking Care Of Things

Bernie always took care of so many things, but now when they went wrong, or something needed doing,

I either didn't know how, didn't have the reach or the strength. In many ways, my time was never my own anymore, and with always feeling that I had to be on guard watching Bernie, I couldn't give time to learning and doing everything.

Fortunately I had a handyman and an auto mechanic who both understood about Bernie and were genuinely helpful. I just came right out and told anyone whose help I needed about his dementia--from the gardener to the painter--and everyone in between.

But mostly, it all fell to me to keep everything going. Some things I could get a handle on, like burning down the house. When I came into the kitchen one morning and saw a fire burning in our toaster-oven, I knew it was old and that something might be wrong with it, so I bought a new one. But when Bernie used the new one, I realized that he got confused with the knobs. If he wanted to make toast, he turned on the oven part, not the toaster part, and then went off and left it. I explained how it worked, but that just made him angry and I didn't want to challenge him because his anger was increasing.

I couldn't have a potential fire every day or a confrontation, so I bought a plain simple toaster and put the toaster-oven in the closet. I also had to put away the fireplace matches he kept moving, he might do anything with them, and it beat calling the fire department.

I replaced the electrical outlets next to our bathroom and kitchen sinks with those that will shut off a turned-on appliance if it should get wet; he might easily put something dangerous in water. There were so many simple things that confused him: earphones on an airplane, opening a TV table, closing a folding chair, filling a pitcher of water, a telephone. We'll never have a portable phone. Pull out an antenna, push the 'talk' button--no way--he'd never learn to do that.

Bernie left the car door open, the trunk open, the dishwasher door down, the garage door up. Kitchen cupboards were always open so you really had to watch your head. He left the yard gate open, or opened it *after* the gardener had left.

One day I went into the bathroom with bare feet and stepped into a puddle of water. He had taken a shower and left the shower door open. I was down on my hands and knees wiping it up, knowing that there wasn't a darn thing on this blessed green earth that I could do about it, and really no way to explain that I sometimes thought I was living in a parallel universe.

Because he could no longer sequence, if I asked him to put water in the dog's bowl, then water the plants on the patio, he'd only remember 'patio,' the last thing I said. He might walk outside and stand on the patio, or he'd water the patio, but not the plants. Or he'd water a few plants, but not all the others.

When I asked him to water the tomato bushes, he asked me where they were. How can someone stand in the middle of his own yard and not see tomatoes growing ten feet away?

My brilliant husband with an engineer's mechanical mind who could fix anything now had trouble changing light bulbs. He couldn't remember whether the globe he was holding was the new one or the burnt-out one, so he'd try them over and over again. Soon he forgot what he was doing, and used bulbs got returned to the closet. I never knew what was what or where. He couldn't even figure out how to open a window!

Letting It Slide

These little things, really of small consequence, happened constantly, but required that I had to redo all the impossible things he'd been so busy with. It further entailed my doing it in such a way that it didn't upset him further and assault his self-esteem.

No one believes that it is possible to lose tomato plants in your own yard, to be unable to change a light bulb or open a window--only breathing could be easier. But that's what dementia does to a person. What it does to those of us who care for them is another matter, and most people just don't believe or understand.

Eventually, as I learned to let things slide, I found that there was rarely anything important enough to take a stand on. Unless there was danger, I just let everything go. I avoided conflicts and battles I knew would never have a resolution. I realized that I couldn't win with dementia, but I didn't lose as often if I just agreed, didn't argue or challenge.

In no time, I developed enough patience to sell, but I couldn't do that because I needed every last shred of it that I could muster daily. And through it all, the important thing was to know what 'important' really meant.

All this aside though, I could see that things were getting very serious. It was obvious that Bernie was declining. I decided to get a second opinion.

♦THREE♦

October 1994

Shingles

Any second opinion would have to wait. I had shingles! Dr. Franklin said it was the worst case he'd seen in all his years of medical practice. I felt like the man who was going to be hung. "If it weren't for the honor of the thing," he mused, "I'd just as soon it was someone else."

An ugly rash covered the left side of my torso and I was in dire pain for six weeks, 24 hours a day without any letup. Nerve endings became flaming piercing jolts and muscles turned into twisted, knotted, smoldering giant pretzels. No shots, no drugs, no salves, no medications could relieve it. And as if the unrelenting pain wasn't enough, it began to affect my thought processes; I was unable to think clearly, to focus on anything. My mind was a constant, terrifying gray fog. Shingles completely sapped every ounce of my body's energy.

When the pain finally went away, I was so weak I literally couldn't walk across the room, so Bernie and I went to a nearby health spa where we'd be in a safe cocoon. I could recoup my strength and Bernie would be taken care of. For two weeks all I did was sleep, then I'd wake up and sleep some more. But it worked. Afterwards I felt fine.

And yes, it is believed that shingles can be brought on by stress. Now, what could have caused that!!

December 1994

A Second Opinion

We went to one of the best neurologists in Los Angeles, but the second opinion was much like the first. When I asked if anything else could be done, he mentioned Cognex, a drug being tested at the University of California Los Angeles (UCLA). In a very small percentage of people, the drug could delay the progress of the disease by about seven months. After that, the patient usually declined again. Maybe, during the delay, something else might come along, although he didn't know of anything.

It could cause liver damage, so the patient had to be continually examined and monitored with blood draws. If liver damage showed up, the patient would be taken off the drug. That didn't make sense to me. Where would we be if the likely damage showed up? Back at square one, that's where. I wasn't happy with the outcome of our visit, but at least I felt better knowing that a renowned expert agreed there really wasn't anything else to be done. I didn't want to leave any stone unturned.

May 1995

UCLA

Six months later, I decided to try UCLA anyway. Who knows? Maybe there was another stone to turn. So with renewed hope, I took Bernie to where we'd finally get thorough, state-of-the-art testing. They'd find out what the problem was and have a course of treatment.

There were several appointments just to consult and a lot of questions for me to answer. Sometimes I was given four or five typewritten pages of questions, other times they were asked orally, dozens and dozens of questions. I tried to be clear and accurate, even when I got tired and emotional. Some of it just hit the wrong nerve.

Bernie's tests included dye injections, being hooked up to machines, things stuck on his head, a battery of blood tests and neuropsychological testing. He was examined physically and memorywise--asked to spell 'world' backwards, to draw circles and triangles, and all the other questions and little games I had come to recognize as standard. We saw several doctors, technicians, and counselors. I was happy that they seemed to be covering all the bases.

Finally our appointment came with the doctor in charge who had reviewed all the findings and would give us a diagnosis. I was excited because now we'd know exactly what was going on.

So, exactly, this is what the doctor said. "Well, we can't say it's Alzheimer's, and we can't say it isn't. But we'll put him in our drug program. I'll have someone call you to make an appointment."

WHAT!

We knew all that before they started testing, and while I knew that uncertainty was the standard diagnosis you get with Alzheimer's symptoms, I wanted more, something tangible. Pull it out of the sky if you have to, but tell me *something.* After all they'd put him through, I expected more, hoped for more, but there was no discussion, no analysis, no nothing.

Now, on the basis of such a vague diagnosis, a flip of a coin--maybe Alzheimer's, maybe not--they wanted him to take an experimental drug that could damage his liver with scant hope of improvement. What was the point of making him feel sick physically on top of his anxiety about just having dementia, much less annoyed with all the appointments and tests?

Although it was Alzheimer's research, everyone at UCLA kept assuring me that they took other dementia patients as well, and that he could be pre-Alzheimer's. Maybe it really would help ward off Alzheimer's, but it was just too big a catchall for me. I couldn't do it.

The doctor had no way of knowing that I already knew about Cognex. He didn't mention the drug by name or comment about any side effects. There was nothing about all the necessary follow-up physicals and blood tests, just that they'd put him in the program, as if it was a gift. But I wasn't about to subject Bernie to any of it. I just wanted to get out. So far, I hadn't heard one word, yea or nay, about constricted blood vessels, being able to improve blood circulation and increase oxygen. No one gave me satisfactory answers to my questions, and maybe there weren't any anyway.

During this time, a polyp was discovered in Bernie's colon, and because he had a family history of colon cancer, it had to come out. Surgery would be in three days and I told the doctor I was going to wait until he was completely recovered to make a decision about the drug program. To think otherwise would be criminal, and besides, my emotions just couldn't handle all of this at once. I said, "No, don't call us, we'll call you." Just like they say in Hollywood.

As we stepped into the hall I knew we'd never come back and Bernie said, "I don't want to be anyone's guinea pig." Obviously, he was well aware of what was going on. I agreed we shouldn't enter the drug program, and told him that was the end of it--but it wasn't.

The next day--THE VERY NEXT DAY--I got a call from someone at UCLA to set up an appointment for Bernie's drug therapy! Why wasn't I surprised? I knew all along that no one was *listening* to me. I had come to the conclusion that they were less interested in Bernie as a patient they could help, than in screening him as a candidate for their research. That may be a harsh assessment, but that's what I came to believe, or maybe they assumed I knew that from the beginning. Either way, it's no wonder we get angry and frustrated--too often, some professionals just don't *listen.*

I'm grateful there is research going on at UCLA and other places. I admire that, wish everyone nothing but success. But in this case, there would be no *long-term* benefit to Bernie, and in fact, could have a negative impact. I wanted to go back to the doctor and say, "Need I remind you? First do no harm!"

Over time, though, UCLA asked us to participate in several research studies for patients and caregivers, and I always agreed, so long as it didn't involve certain medications and was not, otherwise, invasive. Each time they tried again to push him into their Cognex program, assuring me that any liver damage was reversed when the treatments were stopped.

They kept telling me that the sooner a patient takes the drug, the better the chances of success, but so far there wasn't much success in my view. Maybe if some doctor had been more definitive that he likely had Alzheimer's, I'd have felt differently, but they'd float out this iffy idea that Cognex might help patients with dementia as well and it just made me uncomfortable.

I certainly didn't know much about how the brain worked, about neurons, synapses, and other such technicalities, only that it was important for all these little things to keep sending and receiving electrical impulses. But Bernie needed oxygen as well. This was not the program for him.

Still, I made one last phone call to the office of the neurologist who first told me about Cognex and asked, "If your wife had dementia, would you give it to her?" His answer was an emphatic, "No." I felt I was doing the right thing.

(Although Cognex is still available, it is no longer used as a first-line treatment for Alzheimer's.)

"Don't Call Me Caregiver!"

Everyplace I went trying to find help for Bernie, that's what I was called, the 'caregiver.' It drove me nuts. I was *not* a 'caregiver.' In this little scenario, I was the wife, and that's all I ever wanted to be. But no matter how many times I asked not to be addressed as 'caregiver,' that's what it always was.

I was asked to answer the most stupid things, like: "Do you care for your husband to save money?" or "Do you care for your husband out of religious convictions?" Pages and pages of that stuff. Why didn't anyone ask me if I cared for my husband because I had loved him all my adult life? That's the only reason

I can think of. I mean, *really*, who dreams up all that stuff!

Until then, I'd never thought very much about caregivers, but I knew that as a caregiver, so far, I had it pretty easy. Bernie was not physically disabled in any way. He groomed and dressed himself, and if conditions were right, he could make himself a sandwich and something to drink. But that was problematic when I wasn't around, although I was usually around.

I cannot, for the life of me, imagine the physical and emotional drain on a caregiver who has to lift, turn, dress, feed, bathe, medicate, and entertain a loved one, and not only for those with dementia, but for other devastating conditions as well. In millions of homes, tubes have to be checked, injections given, bedpans emptied, bandages applied, things washed and sterilized, special foods prepared, and it's 24 hours a day, every day, seven days a week--24/7--year after year, without respite, and hardly anyone knows and fewer care. "So you're taking care of your father, big deal, didn't he take care of you when you were little?"

Caregiving Is Not For Sissies

No one prepares us to be caregivers. We pretty much fly or crash by the seat of our pants. Success or failure depends on what went on in our lives before--the relationship with the patient, his health, the caregiver's health, sense of self esteem, life style, attitudes, everything. One day someone sticks the label 'caregiver' on you and you're stuck with it. Books have been written for caregivers, articles published, mostly by and for professionals. While some caregiver books have been written by family members, we non-professionals are pretty much left hanging out here alone, except that we don't have the luxury of twisting slowly in the wind. We spin--rapidly--from one crisis to another, like a firefighter rushing to put out one spark after another and another and another and another...

You can think of caregiving on a scale of I to I00. From I to I00, *everything* changes. The relationship between the caregiver and the patient, the socializing, the plans, the activities will all be altered. A child caring for a mother now becomes the parent; a demanding husband taking care of an ailing wife will have to fetch his own beer from the fridge. Passion will become platonic, frustrations for both is a given. The differences on the scale are in how much pressure is on the caregiver, how much care the patient needs.

The cardinal rule of caregiving for patients with dementia is that it is *never* finished. There is *never* any rest for the weary, and caregivers are *always* weary. More than one caregiver has died while the patient lived on for years.

July 1995

Surgery

It was time for Bernie's colon surgery. A counselor at UCLA had told me that I needed to stay with him 24 hours a day in the hospital because you couldn't rely on what he might say or do, he had to be watched. Since I had nothing else going anyway, I asked for a cot to be put in his room for me. I was looking forward to having a few days rest.

When he woke up after surgery, Bernie had no idea where he was or what had happened. In no time at all, he was trying to undo all the intravenous (IV) tubes, pulling and twisting them, looking bewildered, like he was caught in a giant web. I constantly tried to keep his hands away; I was tempted to tie them down. I asked the nurses to tell him to leave the lines alone, hoping their authority would help, but it didn't.

Then he wanted to get up to go to the bathroom. I kept explaining about the catheter, but he didn't understand. When he tried to get out of bed, I asked him what he wanted, and he told me he was looking for the bag the nurse said he needed so he could urinate in it. Again, I explained that the bag was attached to him, indeed, it was filling up, but it still made no impression.

Of course he was in pain, but he insisted that his incision was in his right shoulder when it was on the left side down by his waist. How could he not know where it hurt? When visitors came in, asking how he felt, he pointed to his shoulder every time, said he had a tumor taken out near his collarbone, and no one questioned it! I kept telling the hospital staff that they couldn't trust what he said, but only a few nurses who'd dealt personally with dementia before understood. No one else cared to listen to me, and Bernie absolutely refused to stop tugging at the IV's and trying to get out of bed. I know if I wasn't there, he'd have fallen on the floor, pulling down the IV stand and sprawl tangled in all the equipment.

Each day, Matt came by and stayed with him for a couple of hours. I'd go to the employees' cafeteria, put my head on the table and zone out. Except for those times, I was in that hospital room with Bernie all day and all night. Other people volunteered to stay with him, but they didn't know what they'd be getting into, and I couldn't put that responsibility on anyone.

When Bernie complained about the pain, I'd ring for a painkiller; he had no understanding of how to do that. Then, thankfully, he'd fall asleep and I could get a little rest.

He was doing and saying such odd things--things that I don't want to remember. I was forever on the alert, and not getting much sleep. It was breaking my heart to watch him.

When he could finally get up, we took the IV stand with all its tubes and the urine bag for a walk in the corridor. I called the stand "Gulp," and Bernie thought that was funny, like we were walking a dog. But once he was up and stronger, things got worse. He'd forget he was attached to tubes and try to take out the needle or unhook things from "Gulp." He just got all bollixed up in everything. I kept undoing him, trying to keep everything in place.

Finally his system began working again, he was eating solid foods, the catheter was removed and, with "Gulp" in tow, he could go to the bathroom alone now. I was surprised, then, when he called me into the bathroom, panic all over his face. He was standing with a dispenser of adhesive tape cutting off little pieces and trying to tape the IV tubes to his boxer shorts. He wanted me to help get them all in the right place. Of course it didn't make any sense, taping IV tubes to his clothes, but he was so concerned he wasn't doing it the right way that he was on the verge of tears. The drugs were making his sad mental condition ever more pronounced.

I got him back into bed, assured him he didn't have to tape the tubes, but it was only the last straw in a constant pattern of bizarre behavior that had been tearing me apart for days. I began to see the room literally closing in, getting smaller and smaller by the minute, and I knew I was slipping into deep trouble.

I asked for a private nurse to stay with him, I didn't feel I could leave him alone, anything could happen, but I had to get away. Nothing like this had ever happened to me before. Thankfully, a nurse was there within the hour and I fled home.

Breaking Down

I barely made it into the house before I threw myself on our bed and began to sob. Big, choking, massive sobs that kept increasing while I rolled, screamed, and beat at the bed. These were two years of pent-up tears and they wouldn't stop, couldn't stop. My inner ears seemed to fill up, they were throbbing, I couldn't hear anything, my head was pounding, I was shaking, and still I couldn't stop. I thought my blood pressure would burst through the top of my head.

I was really frightened and I didn't know what to do. Dr. Franklin had recently retired, I had no personal physician, no one to call--and I was so scared. I couldn't come down from the crying jag and the throbbing wouldn't stop.

Then I remembered that Dr. Franklin had sent our medical files to his former partner. I called his office, told the receptionist what was happening to me and asked if I could come in. Much to my relief, she said 'yes.'

I was so grateful a doctor would see me on such short notice. He calmed me down and listened to my story. He, then, a doctor who didn't know me at all, was the one who told me that I had to understand that from now on my health would depend on the state of my husband's health. It didn't seem fair, *wasn't fair,* but I had already sensed that and understood. I assured him that I always took my blood pressure pills, and tried to take care of myself as well as Bernie. But right then, I was simply exhausted, physically and emotionally, and wound way too tight.

He prescribed Xanax, telling me to use it to help me over this rough spot. The problem is, when you're taking care of someone with dementia, there's always a rough spot.

I took half of one, and by the time I got back to the hospital, I was doing better. I had something to eat and went to Bernie's room. He was sleeping. I'd been gone five hours.

The next morning, the last of the IV's were removed and when the surgeon came for rounds, I asked if we could go home early. I thought we'd both be better off there. And so we were discharged--the two of us. We left "Gulp" behind and went home to 'Sophie.'

◆FOUR◆

September 1995

The Control Group

UCLA was researching a new drug, Aricept, costing $400.00 for 90 pills, recently FDA approved, but without the liver damage, and they wanted Bernie to participate. I already knew about the drug, and that it could have other side effects like nausea, diarrhea, insomnia, vomiting and stomach cramps, but that they usually went away.

Private doctors were giving it to their patients, and I'd heard that many of them responded positively, but for a substantial number there was no improvement, no slowing of progression. I didn't know how long the effects might last, it could be a giant step forward, but when I asked about blood flow I got a brushed-off response.

Again they told me they considered Bernie pre-Alzheimer, and while I couldn't challenge that assessment, I told them, truthfully, that I knew he wouldn't willingly take the drug. Later they called back and asked if he would be their control group. He'd have a series of EEG's and the results of his brain activity, without taking the medication, would be compared to those who were taking it. Bernie agreed to that.

I also continued to participate in any number of UCLA caregiver studies. Over the phone, in groups, alone, all sorts of things. Once I asked why they kept calling us. I didn't mind, I wanted to do it, but I was just curious. "Oh," the answer came back, "we want to keep track of your husband to do a brain autopsy in pathology, didn't you know?" No, I didn't know, and I was sorry I had asked, because I was happier before I knew.

"Why Don't You At Least Try The Drugs?"

People asked why I didn't at least try the drugs. If they helped some patients even a little, they might help Bernie. But this is the way I saw it.

Suppose you had a bad cough, something was wrong with your lungs. Your friend had a similar cough that turned out to be pneumonia, and she took penicillin. Would you, then, expect a doctor to give you penicillin? Suppose it's cancer, or emphysema, maybe pleurisy, black lung disease, or some strange infection that doesn't even have a name. Any of these conditions may cause a cough, but just because everyone is coughing, you wouldn't give them all penicillin, or even cough drops. So just because a group of patients all had memory loss, you wouldn't give everyone the same medication.

I'd been told that Bernie's blood vessels, neurons, cells, whatever were withering, constricted, atrophied, dying, or some such thing, and I believed it. I wondered--do these medications affect just the part of the brain that controls short-term memory? Does he have more than one condition? No one could tell me.

Also, I had learned that some medications caused personality changes. That's just what I needed. I had all I could do to handle Bernie's changing erratic personality that I already knew, there was no way I could cope with a 'stranger.' That would not be an improvement for either one of us, and absolutely no one had said that these medications have any long-term positive effect, although I hoped that would soon come about. But, since the pace of each patient's disease can be different, how would anyone know if it was a drug halting the progression, or just an individual's progressing slower than the norm? Well, that's what all the research was for, wasn't it, to answer all those questions?

I'd gone to too many doctors, been given too many opinions. There wasn't a consensus among them. If doctors can't agree what causes this condition, what it is, what to do, or give substantial hope, then by default, we have to make our own decisions. And by substantial, I mean I wanted someone to say that any given drug has helped at least 25% to 35% of the people taking it, and had resulted in *long-term* positive results--at least a few years--and so far I hadn't heard that.

(Today, Aricept is the first drug of choice for Alzheimer's, and it is successful in slowing the progression of the disease in many cases, but certainly not all. Sometimes it is effective for a few years, but at the time I was told, as with Cognex, that it would maybe work for seven months or so. The advantage of Aricept was no damage to the liver. Even if Bernie had taken it, after all my years of experience with him, knowing what I now know, I believe he would have been one of those who would not have benefited.)

November 1995

New Orleans, Louisiana

What If Something Happens To Me?

I had finally settled into an accommodation with Bernie's condition after all the ongoing trauma and accepted that there wasn't anything more I could do for him. No more shingles, no more useless testing, no more surgery, no more doctors, just relax and take each day as it comes, and things had been going along pretty well.

So after Bernie was fully recovered from his surgery, we took a long-awaited group tour to New Orleans. It was early morning in the French Quarter, the weather was glorious, and I was feeling great.

Then, somehow I lost my footing, fell forward, and my forehead went full into a steel post holding up an ornate balcony. I tumbled into the gutter and was lying in the street with everyone gathered around, telling me not to move. I knew I was alright, but it bothered me that Bernie was not kneeling beside me with the others. Instead he was standing back from my feet, silhouetted against an incredibly blue sky, staring down at me with a blank expression, as if he didn't know me. That was so unlike him, it unnerved me to see it. Always before he would have been consoling, caring, concerned. Let me sneeze and he'd bring me hot soup. He'd always been my rock. If I flew off the deep end and crashed, I knew he'd still be there. Now I was feeling abandoned, surrounded by strangers.

An ambulance came to take Bernie and me to the hospital, and I told the group director that we'd meet them in the afternoon, as planned, to continue our tour on a riverboat.

At the emergency room, the ambulance driver told the doctor that I'd been unconscious in the gutter for some time! Really? I didn't know that! They x-rayed my head, revealing a skull fracture. I had to be monitored for 48 hours. No going off down little river tributaries where no medical care was available, I was to stay in the hospital.

Back in emergency, problems were presenting themselves. I kept insisting that Bernie had to stay in the hospital with me. I couldn't leave him alone in a strange city. Admissions kept arguing with me, it was out of the question. Finally the emergency doctor interceded and it was agreed they would put a cot in my room for him. We were reversing what we'd just done only months before when he had his surgery.

All this time, I was getting very uncomfortable. The effects of the accident were starting to set in and I wanted a bed in a dark room to rest, not this elevated gurney under glaring lights and people streaming by making noise and constantly talking. I kept asking for a room without any results. Finally someone from Admissions came down and said that the HMO we had just joined in Los Angeles had no record of me! She told me, "They've been searching and searching, but you're not in their files, Elizabeth."

Elizabeth! Elizabeth! I looked at my wristband, and sure enough, there it was, ELIZABETH. The only other time I'd been identified as Elizabeth was on my birth certificate. Now, thanks to Bernie's dementia, 'Betty' didn't exist because he'd told Hospital Admissions that my name was Elizabeth! What possessed him, I'll never know, but months afterwards it continued to cause all sorts of problems getting medical, financial and insurance records straightened out. So much for my accommodation to his condition. Bah!

But the entire incident made me realize again just how dependent Bernie really was, if not on me, then on someone else. I shuddered at what other horrors might have been if something more serious had happened to me, although a skull fracture and concussion were serious enough, but at least I was still able to think and function. It could easily have been so much worse.

January 1996

"An Apple A Day Keeps The Doctor Away... If It's Aimed Right."

Once I knew what was wrong with Bernie, it would have been great if I could have gone to someone and had it fixed on the first attempt without trying this and that, going here and there, from doctor to doctor, spinning wheels.

Nonetheless I took Bernie to see another neurologist. I wanted to ask his opinion about Aricept and told him everything we'd been through, that I hadn't found anything promising, and I was beginning to feel nothing could be done. Then he asked me, "Well, what do you want me to do?"

Maybe I misunderstood, but it was not an auspicious beginning. If he really wanted to know what I wanted him to do, it was to turn my husband back to the way he was. I knew that was impossible, but rather than be flippant, I said I was hoping he'd have some other ideas; maybe something new had come along and what about Aricept or other new medications.

He interviewed me at length, mostly about Bernie's family, and said he thought he might have Huntington's disease, an inherited illness. You find out if you have the gene through a blood test, which he urged us to do. I told him I'd think about it. He never addressed the issue of Aricept. Another *no listener!*

Before our next visit, I sent away for Huntington's literature, the Guthrie family disease. Knowing Bernie's family as well as I do, it simply wasn't possible that he had it, and if there was no cure or prevention, then I certainly didn't want to know. I'd go nuts every time Debby or Matt said they forgot something.

Besides, I had another idea I wanted to explore. I thought that Bernie's testosterone level might be low. There are just certain masculine qualities that men have, even today's sensitive ones, that seemed to be diminishing in Bernie. I've seen it in other older men, but it's not a sexual thing. Maybe it's normal aging, after all. But, by the same token, I know several men his age or older who still have that masculine presence, the way they carry themselves, swagger, how they present themselves. I'm not talking about some men becoming feminine; it's that indefinable thing that makes the sexes act differently from each other. Also, there had been a recent study that female hormones might help protect older women from getting Alzheimer's. Maybe there was no connection, but it seemed like something worth looking into.

The doctor appeared to dismiss my comments, so I was surprised when he gave me a prescription anyway. I wondered why he didn't have Bernie's testosterone level checked, but he was the doctor. When I took it to the pharmacist, he asked me if I knew that it was an aphrodisiac (wink, wink). No, I didn't, of course. I asked him if it was testosterone. He said it wasn't.

Ah, geeez, life isn't complex enough, now they're giving aphrodisiacs to a 66-year-old man with dementia. Geeez. Just what society needs, another dirty old man. Geeez.

I was vastly annoyed about the testosterone, and really tired of hearing about Huntington's and nothing about my Aricept questions, so I stopped taking Bernie to see him.

We were still dead in the doldrums.

(Now, years later, according to a study published in the February 2004 issue of 'Neurology,' low testosterone levels appear to contribute to neurodegeneration in men with Alzheimer's disease and Parkinson's disease.)

◆FIVE◆

October 1996

Support

I'd gone to a party and, as usual, people asked about Bernie. For all the complaining I did that no one really understood, I could just as easily run into trouble when someone tried. To be honest, I didn't think most people really cared, they were just grateful that it wasn't them. Asking was a courtesy, I've done the same thing. And, in all fairness, what could anyone have done about it anyway.

So I mentioned that a doctor wanted him to be tested for Huntington's but I had decided against it. I was roundly criticized for this attitude. "How can you know what you're dealing with if you don't examine every possibility?" they challenged. Well, the truth is, I thought I knew exactly what I was dealing with, and through no fault of their own, they didn't.

It was then that I decided to join a support group and talk with others who knew where I was coming from. I couldn't keep talking only to Debby and Matt. Bernie was their father--it couldn't be all that easy for them. So I just shut up and let the challenge go unmet. I tried to enjoy the rest of the afternoon.

Group

Oh, no! This was exactly what I feared would happen. I was sitting across the room from two women who were taking turns crying and telling the group about recently placing their husbands. "Placing," that's the euphemism I learned is used for 'putting someone in a home'; and "home" being a euphemism for an 'institution.' It didn't matter what the words were, I could see they were hurting, and I was hurting with them, crying inside for strangers I never knew existed until that morning. As soon as it was time, I was going to leave and never come back. Never! I didn't need this!

"Never Say Never"

Of course, I went back and deliberately monopolized a couple of sessions because I needed some honest answers and Group was the place to get them. I didn't return only for the obvious understanding, compassion and stories I knew I'd exchange with the others; I was also looking for some commonality in the patients and information about meds.

But there wasn't any commonality. None of the husbands were workaholics like Bernie. Two of them had been alcoholics. Most had hobbies, played tennis, golf, cards. Some were mean as junkyard dogs, others were witty, gentle, loving, and none had unusually great stresses. They all had different careers. There were good family men, and others who just wanted to be left alone.

The medications were some that I had heard of, but most caregivers didn't seem to think they brought any significant improvement. One wife swore by the Aricept her husband was taking, but some of the other women who knew him told me that it was mostly her imagination. He had 'improved' at first, but soon was back to his old self and, in fact, was getting worse.

What they told me may have been grim, and there was nothing to hang an explanation on, but I felt that I had received some honest, unfiltered, first-hand experienced information. No one had an ax to grind, a research study, or a pill to sell. I was glad because it helped me feel confident about some of the decisions I'd made.

I went to group for about four months, then dropped out because I was simply tired of hearing my own voice plowing the same ground over and over again every week. But I got a lot more out of those meetings than I ever thought I would and a tremendous amount of valuable tips on how to handle all the impossible situations that keep coming at you. Mostly, though, life had become like living in the middle of a meteor shower. Duck! Sometimes that's all one can do. Duck!

"Yes, We Have No Bananas"

When I was a little girl, it was so much fun, sitting next to my father on the piano stool, legs dangling, singing off key, "Yes, We Have No Bananas," while he played. It always made me happy, but now it made me cry.

I was taking Bernie to adult day care. He didn't object to going, but I had to stay in a separate room the first time or two. There would be music, crafts, lunch, and exercise. I really hoped it'd work. Maybe he'd make new friends, get some interests going.

Through the half-open door where I waited, I could hear his participating in a discussion about a 63-year old woman's giving birth, and he was perfectly lucid, making valid points about the effect it would eventually have on the child.

Soon I heard music and sneaked a peek. That's when I lost it. He was sitting in a circle with the others, like children in kindergarten, this brilliant, loving, handsome man, shaking a tambourine, mouthing the stupid words to that stupid, stupid song, "Yes, We Have No Bananas." I didn't want to see this. I wanted to see him angry, resisting the program, offended that I'd take him to such a place--refusing to participate.

I began backing away from the door, pushing myself into the farthest corner of the room. If there had been a hole under the carpet, I would have crawled in and pulled it down over my head. I couldn't bear to see what I had just seen, and the tears came in overpowering waves, tears that would not be stanched.

Someone was sitting next to me, the program director, talking, but I couldn't understand her at first. Finally her words came clear. "It's not your fault, dear, you shouldn't be feeling guilty." She kept repeating that, handing me tissues from a box, and she wouldn't stop saying it. I couldn't make her stop saying it and I couldn't stop crying.

I didn't feel guilty. Why would she think that I'd feel guilty? I didn't cause any of this. I'd have to be crazy to bring such anguish into our lives, although I could wish that I had such power. If I had that kind of power, I'd undo it all.

It took great effort for me, finally, to stop crying, to tell her the obvious--I wasn't feeling guilty, I was *grieving*. She didn't seem to know what to say. I asked her to leave and she did. It was clear to me, more than ever, that Bernie was embarking alone on a journey where I could never follow. Our life, as we had always lived it, was over--I was grieving.

At lunch break, Bernie found me and said he wanted to leave. So did I. He told me that he didn't want to come back again and I agreed. There were no more tears as I drove away. Not to worry--I knew I wouldn't lack for them in the future.

February 1997

Sacramento, California

"A Death In The Family"

James Agee

Most people close to us really didn't see the changes that Debby, Matt and I saw in Bernie. I can't be certain what they each thought, but I believe there were those who looked a bit askance at me. Their own eyes and observations told them that nothing was wrong. Of course, they only saw him for brief, limited times, that's quite different than being with him 24/7.

Bernie had a niece who lived close to us as she was growing up. We routinely interacted with the family until they moved to Sacramento. When she married, we went to her wedding, praised her new baby and, more or less, kept in touch, seeing each other every few years. Bernie knew her well and she died too young.

There were six or eight of us, family members, who went together from Los Angeles to Sacramento for the funeral. I was glad that so many people who knew us were going to be around, it would make things easier for me. Ever since Paris, I thought travel sometimes made Bernie worse, but I wasn't worried about this brief trip, only a couple of days, surrounded by people he knew well.

Bernie was quiet during the chapel services, the casket was open, but he made no mention of this woman he'd been so close to. He seemed oblivious that we were even at a funeral. For the most part, he seemed to be having a fine time. At the reception later, he told me, "Isn't this a great party," and looking around at all his relatives, continued, "everyone is here."

I didn't have the time nor the inclination to talk a lot about Bernie to his family during those two days, but afterwards some of them told me, "I see what you mean." Nothing unusual had happened, Bernie behaved perfectly well, but being around him for longer periods of time made them see that his seeming normalcy was not all that normal, and if I had asked them to tell me why, what had he said or done, I don't think they would have been able to describe anything out of the ordinary.

"It Is A Man's Own Fault, It Is From Want Of Use, If His Mind Grows Torpid In Old Age."

Samuel Johnson

With all due respect to the esteemed S. Johnson and other sages of his ilk, the time-honored universal belief that 'use it or lose it' is a valid prescription that will keep your mind sharp, is a lot of wishful thinking. We all know of those who can't count with their shoes on, yet they live quite well into their 90's, and other brilliant men and women who, after a lifetime of mental agility, get senile. Go figure.

Over and over again I heard that I had to see that Bernie kept his mind and body active, that this would help his condition. I knew that was not the problem. When I first noticed he was acting funny he was still working in a 10,000 square foot building and spent most of his day walking from one end to the other over and over again. He frequently walked in the neighborhood, or made little jogging circles around the house and yard--it was never in his nature to sit still, and his mind, too, was always active.

Here's the truth--dementia patients have *very* active minds, they 'use it' all the time, just not in a normal way. Before he had dementia, Bernie was constantly devising ways to improve the design of transformers, making drawings and machining parts for one thing or another. He was involved with all the mental tasks of running a business, from knowing his accounts receivable to all the ins and outs of workers' compensation rules and regulations. He read trade magazines. He kept our racecars running--and winning. He never stopped doing all the things that the 'use it or lose it' philosophy considers so important. So how did he 'lose' it?

All along, I was noticing--and dismissing--a change in behavior. He'd come home early from work, although he'd always worked late. He seemed to be at loose ends, and he'd relate incidents or tell me things that didn't really ring true. He'd sit on the couch with his eyes closed and rub his forehead, maybe doze off, or went into the garage, but didn't seem to achieve anything. He lost enthusiasm for his work, but I attributed that to problems with colleagues--and I'm sure there was some of that, but it was only incidental.

What can I say? I noticed, but I didn't notice. I wish now that I had been more compassionate, more understanding, more comforting--but of what? I sometimes think that I let him go through this frightening phase all alone, when I could have held him closer. But why? For coming home early? Most of the time I was glad to see him.

Looking back, trying to piece this all together, I know that his dementia had absolutely nothing to do with his not keeping physically and mentally active. He never willingly gave up any of that. In fact, I believe that he fought incredibly hard against it, as hard as he could.

Doing Stuff

I got Bernie books and magazines, and he'd usually begin reading anyplace in the text, not necessarily at the beginning or where he'd left off, he'd read the same thing over and over. The same with the newspaper, until finally he didn't even make a pretense of reading anymore.

I tried to interest him in jigsaw puzzles, cards, and a variety of games. We took swimming lessons but he never got past splashing with his fingers all spread apart. I signed us up in a gym, and because he couldn't remember how to properly use the equipment I hired a personal trainer. Each session was as if Bernie had never been there before, and after a while he said he didn't want to go anymore.

We went to the senior citizens center for line dancing. The women were all excited about Bernie and when he couldn't seem to get the steps, several offered to show him how. "Stand next to me," one or the other would say, and he'd stand there, but he never got it. He was having fun, but it was embarrassing, and women who wanted him close at first began moving away. He was knocking them around like so many tenpins.

Which brings me to bowling. I signed us up with a league. You wouldn't think it could be so complicated. First I had to see that he got his shoes changed and his ball in the rack--all of which confused him. Then I had to keep track of when his turn was as well as my own. When it was his turn, he might stand anywhere, so I'd have to place him in the right spot. He'd forget to throw the second ball, then he'd forget to sit down and I'd have to lead him to a seat.

Each week, as we approached a different team to bowl, I could see them stiffen, the annoyance in their faces and the tone of voice. No one ever said anything directly, but Bernie was the only one having a good time. I felt I had to stop.

We tried a variety of volunteer organizations, stage plays, car shows, whatever--nothing held his interest and he never asked about going back to any of it.

•SIX•

August 1997

Gorillas In The Kitchen

As a 24/7 stay-at-home caregiver, I long ago learned that there was no way to logically reason with someone who has dementia. In order to discuss something logically, Bernie and I each needed to be on the same mental wavelength, and we weren't, although he thought that we were.

In order to be logical, I had to think illogically. Bernie would be sitting and I'd tell him he needed to change his trousers. OK, he'd say and continue sitting. I'd tell him to stand up and he'd say he was standing. It didn't seem possible that someone would not know whether or not he was standing or sitting, even argue the point, but that's what he'd do. I'd ask if he'd let me help him stand, he'd say 'yes,' then resist my trying to get him up.

I couldn't reason with him, and I couldn't physically pull him up. So I'd have to devise something to make him stand. Maybe I'd ask him to help me move a chair, whatever it took, and as soon as he stood up to do that, I'd grab him before he started to sit again, which wasn't always easy. He'd forget about the chair soon enough.

Trying to get his trousers off while he kept trying to sit down was a real tussle. I'd ask him to undo his belt buckle, and he'd just pull it tighter, I'd pull down the zipper and he'd pull it back up. I'd try to put something in his hands or ask him to hold my shoulders so I wouldn't fall, whatever I could think of to keep his hands off his pants. As the pants started to come down, he'd pull them back up with more strength than I had to pull them down. The more I said 'down' the more he pulled 'up.' Just as he didn't know the difference between sit and stand, he didn't know the difference between up and down, in and out, off and on, come and go, open and shut.

I couldn't reason logically with Bernie, I couldn't argue or fight without making matters worse--he'd just get angry, and I couldn't physically control him because he was so much stronger than me.

It got to the point that if he said there was a gorilla in the kitchen; I'd reach for a bunch of bananas.

Respite

Respite is no small subject when you're a caregiver. Because I'm a night owl, I was up most nights for several hours after Bernie went to sleep. This gave me time to myself, time that I zealously treasured. I could read, do needlework, soak in the tub, whatever, and not have to be concerned about what he was doing.

Bernie and I just got along for the most part and I was getting immune, dismissing the crazy things he did, letting it run off my back. But then I'd come up the driveway and see that he'd pulled the front drapes again in the middle of the day, such a small thing, and I'd get angry. It's daylight, the sun is nice, but he was obsessed with closing the stupid drapes. Without saying anything, I'd fling them open wide, flooding the room in a warm glow, and he'd start explaining why he'd closed them, but I wasn't listening. What was the point?

When this sort of thing built up I'd think about getting away, leaving Bernie with someone who knew, who understood, who cared and could do it--and for that--there was only Matt. Debby would have done it, too, if she was here, but France is France. I told Matt that if I could count on a day or two every couple of months, that would be enough and he agreed he would be there for me.

Some people invited me to stay at their homes while Matt took over, but I wanted to be alone. Being a caregiver means never really being alone, and while I didn't want to always be alone, I just wanted time off, time when I didn't have to answer questions, make decisions, give explanations, make the physical and mental effort to speak.

So Matt stayed with Bernie and I rented a hotel room on the beach. Bernie thought I was staying with a friend in Palm Springs. I went for a long slow walk, looked at all the young families, smiled at lovers, checked out the boats in their slips, and stared at the ocean.

I went bowling and tried to improve my score. Back at the hotel I had dinner, then spent the evening doing embroidery. The next day, at the mall, I had Chinese for lunch and was ready to go home.

About The Tunnel

Painfully, I had been learning that short-term memory loss, dementia, or whatever, was not a benign condition, not at all. And as Bernie changed, I was coming to accept profound, unbidden, pliable changes in myself.

For a long time I had envisioned myself standing alone in a giant empty tunnel, easily big enough for an 18-wheeler, with room to spare. Round, with plain, smooth, concrete walls, its location was someplace underground, but the surface of the earth was not very far above me--maybe there was a park. The tunnel was silent, hidden. Somewhere there was a dim light because I could see. But I couldn't see the end of the tunnel, maybe fifty feet in front of me, just a darkness that completely filled the tunnel round, like a scrim one could walk through, but not see through.

I had no sense of any emotion. I was not frightened, not waiting, not moving, not thinking, just standing--isolated and safe. Whatever I had become bound up in, I knew I would get through it, and I'd be all alone--my inner core was bringing up reserve resources, protecting me.

Unfinished Business

Bernie had fixated on a business associate from thirty years ago and was convinced that person was making money on an invention that belonged to him. There was indeed merit to his thoughts, but it was a dead issue, having been legally settled at the time in Bernie's favor.

I could tell when Bernie began to think about it. He'd get a very dark expression, begin to gnaw on the side of his thumbnail and pace around. Sure enough, after a while he would come to me, and in his most serious manner, tell me to sit down and listen to something really important he had to tell me.

Each time he did this, the story escalated. At first it was just to find the papers, then it was to call our attorney and accountant to discuss it. He wanted to track the man down because he believed he was making millions off his invention. The stories kept getting more and more bizarre, until he even talked about properties we gave him. Of course, there were no properties--never. Evidentially, in Bernie's mind, the legal conclusion was not a satisfactory resolution.

When Bernie told this story it was very convincing. He'd say he had to get a patent attorney, and I'd say that was a good idea, we'll do it first thing tomorrow morning. Whatever he suggested or wanted, I'd respond that we'd take care of it ASAP. I knew that would settle it for the moment, and in the morning--or in ten minutes, he would forget all about it. I also knew it would come up again in a few days or weeks, but so be it.

Bernie usually kept a lot of things about his business to himself. When he had problems with associates, he'd pace around the house muttering and snorting about what he would tell them. Sometimes he'd talk to them in the mirror while he shaved, or possibly he was talking to himself. I don't know, now, who he was talking to, I just assumed it was an associate. I heard it through the closed door, never saw it. At the time, I didn't know that was possibly a portent of things to come.

Or he'd twitch with anger and fury, literally clawing a monkey off his back. These were not involuntary movements; he could control them because he never did them when other people were around. I'd only see it if I walked, unexpectedly, into the room, and then he'd stop.

My suggesting that he try to get help to handle all this anger and stress was futile--although I knew of no one who could help anyway. For a long time, with each adversary either dead or long since gone on to bedevil someone else; he continued to relive everything over and over, again and again. He seemed to be eternally stuck in this quagmire of past events that he had to continually revisit.

It hurt deeply to see someone mentally and emotionally tortured by demons that existed solely in his head. The only thing I could do to make them go away as quickly as possible, the only way that seemed to work, was to agree that they were really there, assure him that we'd take care of it right away--and reach for a banana.

Shadowing And Other Crazy Making

People with dementia are always in your footsteps, watching you, following you, shadowing you--and that's the term used--'shadowing.' You turn around and they're right on your nose. It's understandable, they're frightened. They don't know what just happened or what might come next, and the one they've always been closest to, becomes the one they cling to--like Velcro!

Bernie also forgot where to stand in space. He'd come to the kitchen and stand in the doorway watching me. When I wanted to leave the room, I'd walk to the door and he would just continue to stand in the doorway. It didn't matter how close I came, he just stayed there, filling the doorway so that I couldn't pass. Sometimes, even asking him to move didn't work and I had to physically move him aside, but he still didn't get it. If I were in a hurry, maybe to answer the phone, I'd just push past and then he'd get angry. He didn't understand that others expected him to move, he didn't know what he'd done, and telling him didn't penetrate. He'd lost the ability we all have to simply move out of someone's way.

"The Caregiver From Hell"

There were moments when I'd rage--at Bernie, the disease, the doctors, the insurance company, well-meaning people, the dog, the very air I breathe, and I never knew when it would erupt. For about four years, life had been a trial. Sometimes I felt like I was fighting a lonely battle, and although I had Debby and Matt who supported me and my decisions, I could get really mad. And, yet, I wouldn't have traded places with anyone, not for a nanosecond.

In fact, those years have been among the happiest of my life. They brought great contentment, much joy and a lot of laughter. I came to love and appreciate Bernie in new and surprising ways, I gained great strength, and yet.....

Debby called me 'The Caregiver From Hell,' and probably so did a lot of doctors, only they weren't laughing. I must drive them up the wall. I ask them to make my husband 'all better,' but don't tell me he has Alzheimer's; I have Bernie go through months of testing at UCLA, and then refuse to let him have the medications they offer; I ask a doctor what's wrong with him, and then won't let him be tested.

One day I expected one of them to hand me his stethoscope and say, "Here, you know so much more than I do, you want to make all the decisions and be in charge, you take over while I go out and play golf." Either that, or pretty soon, one of them was going to dropkick me out the front door.

But Bernie couldn't ask the questions, consider the different options and make informed decisions, especially when different doctors said conflicting things. I felt a big responsibility. Someone gave him a pill, I wanted to know what it did and what to expect; someone ordered a test, I wanted to know why. I didn't think I was out of line to ask, and certainly not out of line to question anything that made me uncomfortable.

I just couldn't seem to get a concrete definition of what was wrong. On occasion I called other places, a clinic, another university, but they'd tell me they couldn't take him unless he already had a confirmed diagnosis of Alzheimer's. But I didn't have that, only UCLA's saying they couldn't say.

'Expert' Advice

You'll have to excuse me while I roll on the floor laughing hysterically at some of the 'expert' advice given to people like me. 'Experts' go to school, study, learn from books, take tests, examine patients, get a job in a mental ward, fill in charts, spend years working with demented people and then write a book of advice--usually meant for others in the same field. The problem with professionals is that they go home after ten hours or so of work.

Patient meals are prepared and delivered by someone else. The shopping and kitchen clean up are done by others. Attendants take turns giving baths. Someone else changes linen and does the laundry. Others are busy supervising patient activities. Everyone gets a couple days off each week. Everyday responsibilities do not interfere with taking care of patients.

After work, on weekends, the 'experts' don't have to worry about patient care. They can sleep, clean, cook, and shop; pay bills, do laundry and garden; be with family, talk on the phone, go to the movies, have a romantic interlude--because their demented patients are safely tucked away being cared for by other professionals. I didn't live in that world.

I was on duty 24/7 and emotionally attached to my 'patient' like no professional ever could be. While I was trying to write checks, Bernie would be shuffling the papers around; while I was folding laundry, he was unfolding it; while I was on the phone, I'd know he was up to something. When I was putting groceries away, he was putting lettuce in the microwave and my purse in the refrigerator; while I was in the shower, he'd be outside mucking around somewhere. And I couldn't do everything while he was asleep because I needed to sleep, too.

I also read this advice in the paper--meant, no doubt, to make my life easier. In the kitchen, it directed, keep knives and cooking utensils locked up, put a lock on the refrigerator, freezer and pantry, keep all cleaning supplies locked away, take the knobs off the range and handles off the faucet; keep dishes and glasses locked up, keep all electrical appliances out of reach, well, you get the idea. It's all good advice--NOW COOK DINNER! And remember, while you're cooking, there's a demented adult in the kitchen with you who's helping by picking up knives, hot pans, and moving everything faster than you can possibly keep up with him.

Bathroom, same thing. Lock away all medications, grooming products, cosmetics, bath oils--then take a relaxing bath--while you suspect that somewhere your loved one is starting to repair something that doesn't need to be repaired. And don't forget all those dangerous things in the garage and garden shed. Did you lock them? Are you keeping track of all those keys? And where are those knobs?

'Experts' will always tell you that they understand how hard it is taking care of someone with dementia, but unless they've done it themselves 24/7 for years, they don't know jack.

Yea, well, thanks for the advice, I'll be sure to pass it along.

Whew! I had a good laugh over all of that.

◆SEVEN◆

October 1997

Oxygen Chambers & Chelation Therapy

When I thought about getting oxygen into Bernie's brain, I'd have crazy ideas about sticking a drinking straw in his ear and attaching the other end to an oxygen tank, until finally something concrete occurred to me. I'd put him in an oxygen chamber!

I also did a lot of research on chelation therapy. No doubt it depends on the cause, but many dementia patients have found it successful. Knowing that it cleaned out arteries, I thought it might work on Bernie's constricted blood vessels. I didn't know at the time that they were, in reality, twisted not just constricted. We went to a clinic over an hour away that offered both treatments.

We were also given vitamins and supplements, all sorts of things that were supposed to help his condition. The next morning I gave the pills to him and within 15 minutes he'd upchucked the whole mess. I decided I'd better pay closer attention to what I was doing and divided them into smaller groups. I only gave him a couple new ones every few days so that, if he had a problem with any of them, I would know which ones were causing it. After that, he easily tolerated everything.

Since the treatments would go on for some time and take several hours a day, it would be easier if Bernie stayed in a nearby licensed group home for people who needed care. Bernie's room had twin beds and I was told that I could stay overnight whenever I wanted to at no extra charge, which pleased me. I decided to stay three days a week with him then go home myself for four days.

Although Bernie was OK with the treatments and enjoyed all the socializing, he didn't like it when I left him alone at the home. I kept explaining that it was only temporary, but he always wanted to come home with me.

Another man, Joseph, was also staying there. I was told that he also had dementia, maybe Alzheimer's, and was OK walking around until he fell and broke his hip a month before. Now he was in a wheelchair. Still quite handsome, he didn't look his 72 years. But he was really mean. He hit anyone who came near him, even knocked out one of the owner's teeth! He wouldn't eat, and I never heard him say anything. When I was there, I'd pitch in to help with the other residents, but when I tried to feed Joseph, he raised his fist at me every time I came close, so I stopped.

Within a very short time, however, Joseph was confined to his bed, and I was told that he would die in a matter of weeks. He was failing fast and no longer came to the table. I had no idea what was wrong with him, unless it was just his brain shutting down his body, although he still looked relatively healthy. I didn't see any IV's. Obviously, someone in his family had made a decision. Maybe there was nothing else to be done for him. I didn't know and I didn't ask.

"9-1-1"

The call came at 5:30 in the morning, waking me from a sound sleep. Bernie's voice was low, quavering, "I'm dying, I'm dying--you have to come and get me, I'm dying." And he meant it, I knew he meant it, but I also knew he wasn't dying. "Call Matt, call Matt. You have to come and get me, I'm dying."

For several days I'd been getting calls from him, each one more intense. The phone at the home was attached to the FAX machine and I knew he couldn't figure out how to use it by himself. I didn't think anyone got up at 5:30 to place the call for him, which is what they always did when he wanted to call me.

I hated to wake up Matt, but I had to. I didn't know what I might find when I got there, and I wanted support if I needed it. Before I left the house though, I got another call from the captain of the emergency medical response team. The 'who' of the 'what'? I didn't know what was going on, but the captain told me that he was confused. Yea, right, tell me about it, and as Matt later said, 'get in line.'

The captain was confused because he said he couldn't find anything wrong with Bernie and didn't see any need to take him to the hospital. Oh, his pulse was a little fast, but otherwise he was perfectly fine. He wanted to know if Bernie had any heart conditions, and I told him about his heart murmur. We agreed he didn't need to be hospitalized.

When Matt and I arrived, Bernie was standing in the entry hall waiting, his bag packed, and a smile on his face like a kid with fresh spun cotton candy. In spite of my seeing him so often, all he wanted was to be with me--constantly. So I brought him home. He was completely happy then, his old self--except for the dementia.

This is how he did it without knowing how to use the FAX, but with whatever memory of phone use he still had. He hit the 'O-operator' button and had the operator place the call to me; he still knew our phone number. After he spoke to me, he hung up, hit '9-1-1' and told them he was dying, that he had chest pains and shortness of breath--maybe he did if he was frightened, or maybe he just said 'yes' if they asked him those questions. Within minutes there was an ambulance, a fire truck and a police car--all rolling up, sirens screaming, waking the whole neighborhood, getting everyone up in arms.

I wouldn't be surprised if it weren't all a matter of transference because of Joseph. No doubt he heard people talking about Joseph's dying and it wasn't unreasonable for Bernie to think that this was the house where people died and he wanted out.

There's no question that Bernie truly believed he was dying, but below is a section of the EKG they gave him. Look at it. That straight line with all those firm even peaks at equally spaced intervals--everyone should have such an EKG!

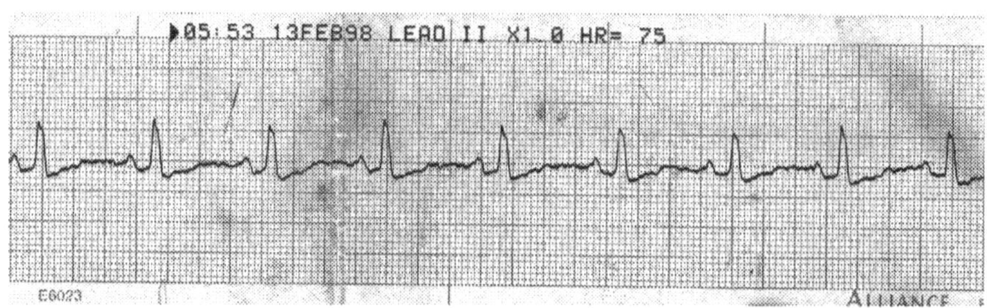

Didn't I tell you that people with dementia have very active minds? Afterwards, he didn't remember any of it, denied it all, and he was being truthful.

In spite of all the critics, I found oxygen chambers and chelation therapy to be perfectly safe. But while they made Bernie feel better, they really didn't help, so I stopped. In my research, I'd heard from more than one source that many doctors use chelation for themselves and their families but dare not say so publicly. I have no idea if that's true, but it wouldn't surprise me one bit.

Getting Battered

All day long Bernie never let me more than three feet away from him. At night I couldn't sleep, so I'd get up to do the crossword puzzle and he'd be right there with me. I'd just let him sit, but that didn't work. He kept glaring, pacing, then he'd decide to get dressed. At 2:00 in the morning, he was going for a walk! He'd be half in pj's and half in street clothes. In and out, over and over, storming throughout the house until finally, one night, I decided to do something I'd never done before in my life.

I'd never given prescription medication to anyone it hadn't been prescribed for. But this time I checked my drug book for any interactions and, since there weren't any, I gave him half of one of my Xanax pills. Thankfully, it calmed him and I got us back into bed, curled up next to him and sweet-talked him to sleep.

Before 7:00 a.m., he was at it again. He was furious with me for sleeping with other men! Where did *this* come from? Defending myself against such nonsense only made him angrier. Then he began weeping about my breaking up the family, how much he loved me, how frightened he was. When he first talked about being frightened, I thought it was because he knew he had something wrong with his mind--but, no, that's not what he said frightened him. What frightened him was losing me. I kept reassuring him that I wouldn't leave him, and that had always been true, but now something new was in the mix--it wasn't my leaving him, it was his driving me away. He wouldn't give me any space, it was well beyond shadowing. I could barely breathe. I felt the noose getting tighter and tighter by the hour.

Every fifteen minutes, all day long, it was 'I love you,' 'you're so beautiful,' 'I'm afraid I'll lose you.' He was literally *stalking* my soul, and I couldn't get away, which made me think about the unthinkable.

I remember when I first sat with Debby and Matt to discuss our situation, I said--and meant it--that I'd just keep Dad at home with me and we'd go on like we always had--so he forgets some things sometimes. I didn't see any problem. But that was another world, and I didn't live there anymore. I couldn't continue like this much longer.

I was alone with him almost all the time--being badly battered mentally and emotionally. If he realized what he was doing to me, he would have certainly stopped, but I knew he couldn't help it. And even though he wouldn't knowingly hurt me for the world, I was still being battered, and it was still taking its toll.

I'd do anything I could to help him, to help us, and as much as I still loved him, even more than ever, I wasn't the type to willingly leap on my husband's funeral pyre. Matt told me, "Mom, please take care of yourself. Deb and I talked about it, and we don't want to lose you to the same disease." They'd gone together to a lecture about Alzheimer's without even telling me, so they were learning more and more, objectively and personally, all the time. They saw enough and knew enough to know that losing me, too, was a possibility. People don't understand, but it happens, too often the caregiver goes first.

"The Thing"

Sometimes I wonder how I am going to write this, I can hardly think about it, but I feel compelled to tell about 'the thing.'

Bernie woke me at 3:00 a.m., one morning. He wanted to tell me something--but then he didn't--and then he did--he couldn't decide. Instinctively I knew that I didn't want to hear it, hoping he'd go back to sleep, but he was too restless. Finally, he told me.

"I found something," he whispered, "I found something. I don't know if I should tell you."

Oh, God, I thought, oh, God, I don't want to hear this--whatever it is, I don't want to hear it. I don't want to hear it. Other than knowing it was all in his mind, I wasn't sure where it all happened--where it was that he 'found something.' It seemed like it had been lying on the garage floor.

"It was red," he continued, forming his hands as if describing a grapefruit. "It was red and meaty and it could think on its own. It could think all alone, without any help, it could think on its own."

I could barely hear him, he spoke in such a hoarse, broken whisper. "I don't know if it was ev-- if it was ev--evi--"

"No," I told him right away, because I knew what was coming before he even said it. "No, it's not evil. See, I'm here, 'Sophie is here in her bed, and Matt's in his house. No, it's not evil, I'm sure of that."

He continued restless for a while longer. Finally I gave him half a Xanax and he fell back to sleep. But I laid in the grip of the silent darkness all around us, watching moon shadows flit on the wall and across his face. I didn't know if he'd had a dream, an hallucination, or if it even mattered. To my mind, he had conjured up his thinking brain and 'found' it separated from him. It could think by itself without him, without his control--and it *was* evil.

◆EIGHT◆

March 1998

What If Something Happens To Me--Again?

Well, it did--again!

I didn't feel right, that's the only definition I can give, I didn't feel right. I had a horrific stomachache, my abdomen was twisting and cramping, but then it would go away and come back a couple hours later. I thought it might be food poisoning, any organ, female or otherwise, but it kept going away. I read my medical book and it wasn't specific enough about abdominal cramps, but it did say if it was an appendix, you could safely wait 12 to 24 hours. I didn't have a fever, although I had a few chills, no vomiting, and the pain was not consistent or localized, just my entire trunk.

All this time Bernie had been at me again about sleeping with other men. Over and over and over again and again--he was absolutely over the edge. I kept pleading with him to leave me alone, I was so sick, but he'd have none of that.

Finally, in such excruciating pain that I was rolling on the floor in a fetal position, I called Matt. Something was terribly wrong and I was unable to drive myself to the emergency room. I couldn't take an ambulance or a taxi because I had to have someone with Bernie all the time, so once again it had to be Matt.

"This Is Like *Deja Vu* All Over Again."

Yogi Berra

At the hospital they weren't sure at first what was wrong. My blood work showed an infection, they just didn't know where. The pain had completely subsided, I was feeling fine. After more tests, exams, poking, consulting three different doctors, they finally determined it was my appendix. My symptoms were atypical, but that's what it was--and it's not supposed to happen to people my age--that's what it said in my medical book. They were not impressed with my book, and so I was being prepped for emergency surgery. It was *déjà vu* all over again, except that this time it wasn't New Orleans and Matt was there to take care of Bernie.

But just like in New Orleans, Bernie became the focus of everything. I was being asked all sorts of questions and about who would care for me at home. Bernie and Matt were standing next to me, and Bernie was asked if he would do it. "Sure," he said, but I told them 'no' because of his dementia. At that, the emergency room doctor ran off to find a handbook about caring for people with dementia. Dammit! Here I was, getting ready to be sliced open like a Thanksgiving turkey, and the doctors were talking about Bernie's dementia. What more did I have to do to get away from it? Was there never again going to be a moment's peace--just for me?

What I thought would be a simple little scar and a couple days in the hospital turned out to be a big long scar and really major, because the appendix had ruptured. Otherwise I was healthy, and by the third day, the surgeon said I was doing fine physically, except that 'something' seemed to be wrong with me. When I told her that I couldn't go home, that my husband wouldn't understand or give me any peace, she said she'd send the social worker up to see me.

"Oh, no, don't do that," I said. "I've seen all the people I care to see about this, I just have to decide what I'm going to do." Nonetheless, in a couple hours the social worker was at my bedside. Again, dementia was intruding. There was no escape. I couldn't even have surgery all to myself.

As a captive audience, I had to listen to the social worker's spiel even though I told her, emphatically, that I didn't want to hear it. But she was so pleased with being able to 'help' me, like so many others, she didn't *listen*. She left pamphlets about stress and grief, and a booklet on elder care on my bedside table, all of which I knew I'd never read. But, who has the strength to argue? Why won't everybody just go away and leave me alone! I tried to sleep.

"Amen" In Any Language

Later that day, two very elegant, regal black women stood outside my open door. One wore a beautiful golden brocade outfit, the other dressed as if for a very special occasion. They were obviously discussing me, then came into my room.

"Would you like us to pray for you?" I didn't hesitate for a moment. Whatever their religion, whatever their motivation, I was ripe for it. My mother always said 'a blessing is better than a curse' and she was right. I figured it couldn't hurt. Now on either side of my bed, each holding one of my hands so tightly I thought they'd stop the circulation, they said their prayers and asked that I be blessed in the name of Jesus. Amen. I actually believe that some of their physical strength passed into me.

Within ten minutes a Rabbi was in the room. "Would you like me to pray with you?" Yes, I told him immediately, you bet I would. And so he, too, prayed for me, in Hebrew and in English. Amen. With that, I figured most of the bases were covered. Given the situation, and in my condition, I was available for anyone or anything. I needed all the prayers and blessings I could get, thank you very much. Amen.

Changing Gears

I realized how helpless I was and knew that I couldn't go home to my own bed, so I went to my sister's house for a few days. Matt took off work to care for Bernie, and we devised a plan of deceit. He'd keep Bernie as distracted as possible and I'd call home two or three times a day to report on what the doctor said and how I was improving, but tell him that I couldn't have any visitors. It gave me time to rest and recover my strength.

When I saw the surgeon post-op, I asked her how serious it had been. She said it was *that* serious, I could milk it for all it was worth, and so I did.

After my appendectomy I had a lot of quiet time to think--not that I could, or even wanted to do anything else--but it was as if my frantic life had come to a screeching halt. Stop for a minute, Nature was telling me, pay attention to what's really going on here. In the past five years, since Bernie was diagnosed with short-term memory loss, I'd had a severe case of shingles, a concussion and an emergency appendectomy. It's not that I live under a lucky star, but this was not like me. I wouldn't go so far as to say that my surgery was a blessing in disguise, but I did think it made me stop and take stock of our situation.

I knew, once and for all, that I had to make arrangements for Bernie's care if I was unable to do it anymore, for whatever reason. I began phoning care facilities. I wasn't ready to place Bernie, but I wanted to have a few possibilities to at least tell Matt about, just in case, because he'd be the one it would all fall to.

As for Bernie, he was just delighted when I came home. He never once asked about my surgery or how I was feeling, he forgot immediately where I'd been and why. He was just so happy that I came back. I could have hit him!

♦NINE♦

April 1998

Accusations

El Nino was savaging the Southland. Dozers were laboring away in Malibu, Laguna was sliding toward the sea, bluffside homes were tumbling like matchsticks, and I was snug in my bed as the gray dawn broke through the blinds, safe on the dull flatlands, content to have my plants and lawn getting fresh rainwater. I loved the rain--not the flooding, of course--but the sound of it gurgling down the rainspout, splattering on the skylight, rivering down the patio bricks to the driveway, misting my windows. But the best part about rain, the very best part, was savoring the coziness of my bed when half asleep. I wasn't prepared, then, for the glare of the bedroom light jolting me fully awake.

"Honey, turn off the lights," I muttered. "Turn 'em off yourself," Bernie flung back at me. Oh, great, I thought. The day had barely begun and he was awake, ready to accuse me again of all manner of wretched things. He *never* turned the lights on when I was asleep, *never*. He'd always been so quiet in the mornings. I never heard doors open, drawers close, no lights--and now--this!

His hostility was palpable; his eyes bore holes into me. "How can you?" he growled. "How can you sleep with other men? Why are you doing this, breaking up our marriage? When are you leaving? Were you even going to tell me about the divorce?"

It wasn't bad enough that he was waking me up, but I had to listen to all this garbage. There was no way I could get these delusions out of his head. Of course, I wanted to fight back, yell at him, tell him how stupid and hurtful he was to me--but it would be useless.

How could he accuse me of such things? Although part of me was thinking, 'from your mouth to God's ear,' I certainly could have used the diversion.

Honestly, I was well beyond anger, so I did the only thing I knew to do, the only way I knew to calm him, distract him. Again, just like I'd done so many times before, I told him, "I'm sorry you feel that way, honey. Come here, sit beside me, you know I love you, come here." And I did love him, that's what hurt so damn much.

He sat on the bed beside me, then laid his head on my chest and told me how much he loved me. He let me stroke his head, soothe him, tell him again and again how much I loved him, how I wanted to be with him. He began to cry. "I need help," he kept saying. I agreed and said that's what I was trying to do. I hadn't given up, but I didn't know where else to turn.

Finally he turned off the light, got back into bed and held me until he fell asleep. If only the rain would wash away all my sorrow and tears, but nothing could change the course of this relentless onslaught engulfing us.

Maybe This Will Help

I decided to write a note for him to keep in his wallet. He could look at it whenever he wanted to. He kept saying that I'd left him, even though I was right there in front of him all the time. The note read, "Bernie, I am not leaving you." When I saw that he had carefully spread it out on top of his dresser, I felt pretty good, believed he was reading it, reassuring himself that I was still here. But then he put it on the kitchen table and added at the bottom: "YOU DID LEAVE." Below is the note, exactly as we both wrote it.

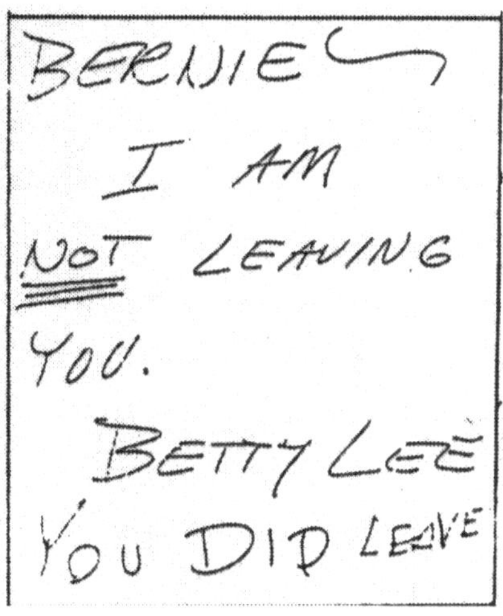
BERNIE
I AM
NOT LEAVING
YOU.
BETTY LEE
YOU DID LEAVE

Denial Denied

You know, all along, no matter what I've written, or said or did, I knew what I knew. Sometimes I was whistling past the graveyard, and I knew that. I wasn't a pathfinder on this journey. I'd seen it made by too many others, heard too many stories to think there was a magic bullet somewhere, I was just stumbling around in the dark. Still, one keeps trying, maybe not hoping exactly, but there's always a 'maybe' isn't there? How did one stop searching for an answer anyway? When did you know that there was nothing more around the next corner?

So where were we? I didn't know what I was doing anymore. I was to the point, though, that I really had to consider something drastic. I'd just about made up my mind. Was I going to wait around until he struck or killed me? I didn't think he really would, but who knew, no one could give me any guarantees--and it has happened to others.

♦TEN♦

April 1998

Dead & Dying

When Bernie called '9-1-1' and told them he was dying, I thought it was partly transference because he knew that the other man, Joseph, was going to die. I didn't pay all that much attention to it. I thought it was a clever ploy to get back home and his resourcefulness pleased me.

But more and more he talked about his own death. Sometimes he would rage at me that he was dead, he had no future, there was nothing to do, nothing he even could do, he was dead, dead, dead. And he'd begun to tell me that he simply would not go into an insane asylum, he'd fight with all he had in him to keep out of an insane asylum, he simply wouldn't go to one--period. In fact, I didn't even know where an insane asylum was, but I did know about assisted living facilities. I told him, promised him, he'd never go to an insane asylum--and he never would, that was for sure. However, that didn't mean he wouldn't have to go someplace else, especially if something happened to me.

He'd very lucidly, clearly talk about our finances. He said he didn't think he had much longer to live and he was concerned about how I'd make out. He wanted to still take care of me. I didn't know what was in his head about dying, but something was definitely there. Whether it was a premonition or not, I couldn't say. I told him we were going to be OK financially, what else could I say? I said we'd be OK even if one or both of us had to go into a home--it was a chance to plant a seed--although I knew he'd forget, but I planted it anyway.

Terror

I went on a few errands and was gone less than two hours. I never worried about leaving him for a while. But this time it was different. When I came home his face was so frightened, so full of terror, I'd never seen it like that. I was afraid to ask what was wrong. Truly, I thought someone had died.

"I thought I lost you," he cried, "I thought I'd lost you, I was so frightened, so scared. You were down by the border in your car and the other cars----." I couldn't follow what he was saying, nothing made sense, I certainly wasn't near the border, nothing had happened.

I wrapped my arms around him and he was trembling, but not like any ordinary tremble, I swear I could feel each cell in his body shaking, slamming into each other, all but bursting through his skin. I couldn't believe his sheer terror.

Usually, I'd make some silly remark about looking for me in the 'Lost and Found,' but I knew I couldn't pretend that I was a misplaced wallet; this was too deeply felt to make light of. So I just held him, soothed him, until he calmed down. I knew then that I'd never be able to leave him alone again. I saw that he had our personal phone book open. Obviously, he'd been calling people, looking for me, alarming everyone. I had to get someone to spell me.

He was completely opposed to that, of course. When I mentioned I was going to get a male companion for him on occasion, he was furious, he didn't want any other man in the house, he was adamant. But Matt couldn't be available all the time, and I couldn't stay with him 24 hours a day, I had to have some relief. Even if he didn't have dementia, 24 hours a day with the same person and no one else was not my idea of the best situation, although I recognized there are those who would be very happy with it. We spent a lot of time together, a lot, but the main problem was that there wasn't anything much we could do together. It was impossible even to have a rational conversation.

He had to always be so close to me that I couldn't do anything by myself. And he never stopped gazing at me, sometimes with such awe that I thought he expected me to levitate. Other times it would be a sappy grin like a teen-aged boy who has just discovered that girls have breasts. Don't look so dopey, I wanted to tell him--and sometimes did.

But then there were all the piercing glares and almost continual horrid accusations. It was getting to be a little much--unrelenting verbal and emotional abuse. I was learning exactly what unabated hectoring was, and to be on the receiving end was just not a lot of fun. Not even when it was done by someone you loved and you knew he couldn't help it--or maybe that made it worse.

"Will You Marry Me?"

You'd think after all the yelling about my getting a divorce and sleeping with other men that Bernie would have wanted to be rid of me, but that's not what happened. Instead, he kept asking me to marry him. The first time it happened, I thought he meant one of those vow renewal ceremonies. The idea of planning such an event was out of the question. I'd have felt very uncomfortable standing up in front of people and renewing vows that I would no longer make. I still loved Bernie, still wanted him in my life, but truthfully, knowing what I know about dementia, I'd never marry him now.

He asked me if we'd ever been married and I showed him our wedding album. It was as if he was seeing it for the first time. He'd forgotten our wedding, and I knew that was a bad sign, a sign of further deterioration. He routinely asked me to marry him. I always said yes, we'd get married the next morning. He'd get so happy, and go on about how jealous everyone would be that I was going to marry him.

He carried it to an extreme. When I said I'd marry him, he began planning the wedding, talking about who we'd invite, saying that we'd have to tell the children that they would be legitimate and wouldn't that surprise them. Indeed it would! He wanted to know if I'd ever been married before, and when I said 'no,' he was ecstatic that he was so lucky. He told me, "I've known you since grammar school and I can't believe I've waited so long."

He maneuvered me into the corner of the couch and leaned so close I couldn't focus my eyes. He began kissing me and talking about seducing me after we were married, staring at me, telling me how beautiful I was, and how lucky he was. My emotions were simply overpowering, I couldn't stand watching it--and it was as if I were watching--I was being torn apart by what was happening, his joy, his glee were so genuine, but it was crushing something inside of me. I closed my eyes, tried to move my head away, but he was too close to me. Finally, barely able to breathe, I asked him to sit beside me, and he did, discussing our wedding, while I took in deep gulps of air and tried to gather myself together.

Where was he now, I wondered? He was living somewhere 50 years ago, completely unaware that it was a half-century down the road. And he'd forgotten it, at least part of it, at least for now. But he was so happy--practically slaphappy.

So now I had a new worry. If he couldn't remember his own wedding, what did that mean? Further regression? Was it only a matter of time until he couldn't remember me, the children, our life together?

Don't answer that!

"Till Death Do Us Part"

Society argues a lot about life and death--when it begins--how it should end. Growing up it was pretty cut and dried to me. Dead was dead. Today it's all different. If someone is brain dead, are they really 'dead'? If you transplant his heart into someone else, have you murdered him? If his heart lives on, can he be truly and completely dead? What about people who are in irreversible comas, only kept alive by machines. If machines are keeping you alive, would you otherwise be completely and truly dead? Well, don't look to me for any answers, I had a different concern.

There is no question that I was still physically attracted to Bernie. But it could never be the same because the essence of his being--that undefined part of us that is not physical--no longer existed. Well, sometimes parts of it did, but essentially it was gone, and with it, in no small measure, was our marriage.

In many ways I treated him as a small child; distracting, diverting, shielding, contriving, guiding, cajoling, whatever it took. The difference was that children learn; adults with dementia really can't, it just gets worse and worse.

We were two people living in the same house, sleeping in the same bed, eating together, but that doesn't make a marriage, does it? The dilemma is this: What is your status when your marriage dies before your spouse? Can 'till death do us part,' also mean the death of the marriage, or was it only specific to the death of your partner?

The answer didn't really matter, I wasn't going to leave either way, it was just something to think about.

Ripping My Heart Out

When someone borrowed Bernie's car and left it badly parked at an angle out front, he told me he was going to go outside and straighten it. Of course, he wasn't supposed to drive, his license had been lifted long ago, fortunately with his understanding. Since there were no other cars parked nearby and I didn't think he'd drive away, I decided not to stop him.

Inside the house, I stood next to 'Sophie' and the two of us watched him from the front window. He sat in the car, touching and moving all the knobs and buttons on the dashboard. The windows went up and down, and I saw the hand brake between the seats pulled up and let down several times. I saw him sitting there the way I'd seen him a thousand times before, in the driver's seat, in charge of his life, knowing just what to do.

Many times he'd drive up to the house as I was leaving on some errand and we'd smile and wave; maybe stop for a moment, lower the window and I'd call, "I'll be back in 15 minutes"; or we'd arrive home at the same time, and go into the house together. Sometimes he'd pull up behind me at the nearby stop sign and toot his horn. I'd see him in the rearview mirror, put my hand out the window and wiggle my fingers at him as I drove off.

How did all those mundane meetings that I'd never given any thought to before become such precious memories? Watching his fumbling with something that had always been second nature only opened the water works in my eyes. What was he thinking? Did he think about his never being able to drive again, about all the loss that meant? Or maybe he was pretending he was driving, the way a child sits in a car and imagines. Finally, I couldn't bear to watch him sit there anymore. Just how many ways can my heart be ripped out of my chest? Shaking it off, I went outside to guide him in straightening the car, leaving 'Sophie' alone to watch us through the window.

"Mommy"

You make the mistake over and over again of thinking things are getting better, it's not all that bad, but it's only to lull you into a false ease, to catch you off guard so that when another blow comes you are not well prepared, and that night I was struck again.

Bernie was acting really well, no problems, he ate a good dinner but then was tired, anxious to get into bed. I was tucking him in, leaning over and gave him a kiss. He had the sweetest smile for me and said, "Thank you, Mommy."

Oh, God in Heaven, what the Hell am I supposed to do? Ice water was running through my veins. I had the strangest feeling that I was my mother-in-law looking at my husband as a child. In an odd way it was very insightful into the way his childhood had been, the kind of mother she was, but I didn't know what to do with those emotions, there was no place to store them.

♦ELEVEN♦

May 1998

"I Am The Lord Thy God, *Dementia*
Thou shalt have no other Gods before Me."

The First Commandment
Exodus, *The Old Testament*

One day I had no one to stay with Bernie so I took him with me to the doctor when I went for a check-up and left him in the waiting room. I was OK, no problems--just keep up the blood pressure medications--and I thought that was that. But at the nurse's desk, she said my husband wanted to talk to the doctor. She didn't know why and neither did I, but we were ushered into his office.

Bernie came right out and asked him, "What can be done so that we can have intercourse?"

Damn! I was furious; tears of anger were pressing the back of my eyes. How dare he! This was MY physical, MY body, MY time. Not only was he taking over MY medical appointment for himself, but he was doing it without any prior discussion, just springing it on me--and on the doctor--without any warning.

Of course, I knew it was the dementia; Bernie would never normally do such a thing. The doctor looked at me and I was barely able to talk. I do everything, everything. I take care of everything, the finances, insurance, the driving, the car, his medications, everything in the house, dealing with repairmen, the yard, his doctors, meals, seeing that he eats his food, showers and shaves, take him for his haircuts, all the shopping, the laundry, remind him to feed 'Sophie,' see that she gets bathed and to the vet, every stupid thing, and now I'm expected to deal with *this!* I was--I was--offended. I mouthed a reminder to the doctor, 'he has dementia.' Of course, he knew that and told Bernie that he should make an appointment to discuss it later; he didn't have time right now.

By the time we left the building, Bernie had forgotten all about it and never mentioned it again. But I was so angry that dementia had intruded into my private space again, that my blood pressure was probably flying on high.

Because my husband had dementia, I was continually subjected to endless absurdities that were impossible to resolve. It was hard to take care of myself as well as him, to monitor my blood pressure, to see my doctor, or whatever else I wanted or needed, maybe do *something* else, think of *something* else just one more time in my life before I die, but *everything* always took a back seat to dementia, and Bernie just went blithely along.

When we were in the hospital in New Orleans with MY cracked skull, home with MY appendectomy, at a rest spa to recover from MY shingles, the thing that took the most time, consumed most of my energy was this hateful dementia. I'm telling you--I had no life of my own anymore. When I die, if I don't do something about it now, it will take over my eulogy, and I don't want it mentioned at all, not in any way, shape, fashion or form. Period!

Here are my instructions to anyone who may read this: ABSOLUTELY NO MENTION OF DEMENTIA IS TO BE MADE AT MY FUNERAL--UNDERSTAND--ABSOLUTELY NONE! I've already spent enough of my life with that monster, I won't have it intruding on my death--it's *my* death and mine alone. If anyone should even breathe the word during that time, I promise I will come back to haunt you--and it won't be pretty. You bet I was resentful!

The Psychiatrist

Still looking for something else--anything--I took him to a psychiatrist. This would be a new approach. Maybe he could get a better handle on things, try some different meds.

The first comment he made when I told him how long Bernie had dementia, was to say, "You've certainly lasted longer than most." The thing was, on occasion, Bernie could be so normal, anyway for a few hours, so it wasn't every minute impossible.

Bernie had started to stay awake at night and walk through the house. Or he'd sit on the edge of the bed for a few minutes, then lie down again, then sit, then lie down. He did it countless times. He'd get partially down and then rise up again--he'd forget in the middle of the action which way he was going.

He was also getting more and more angry, there's no blaming him for that. And while I felt relatively safe, I was never all that 100% certain what he might do, especially when he started in on my sleeping with other men. And then there were other delusions.

"When did you last see Guillaume?" I asked him that in front of the doctor because I knew he'd have a weird response. Bernie said that Guillaume was his nephew, working somewhere down south, or east, in Palm Springs or Mission Viejo, or sometimes at the local sandwich shop, the kitchen in the bowling alley. Everyone liked him; he was such a little hustler, doing such a fine job. Guillaume, of course, was our 13-year-old grandson going to school in the Pyrenees.

After telling several other astonishing tales, the doctor prescribed something to help him sleep and control the delusions. But the next morning Bernie was at it again about other men. He was so worked up, his body rigid, his face red and contorted, fists clenched. Finally he kicked the screen door, really hard, flailing it open.

Since the medicine only increased his agitation and he was still awake all night, after a week or so I stopped it. Xanax was more effective. I tried to keep him awake during the day, but I think it made things worse, besides I couldn't be at him every minute all day. And, I kept falling asleep during the day because I was sleep deprived during the night. Sleep deprivation is the way prisoners are tortured, and I wasn't ever going to be released. For someone who rarely went to bed before midnight, I was zonking out by nine or ten, and finding it impossible to function normally.

I told the psychiatrist about his escalating anger, and he told me that if Bernie hit me to call the police and to always look for an escape route when I was alone with him. I couldn't imagine something like that! No one could live that way, no one should have to live that way. I didn't think he'd hit me, but who knew?

I had no clue where this was all going to end, but I can tell you that I was exhausted! You know when you feel like you're between a rock and a hard spot? That would be a lot more comfortable than the spot I was actually in. I was thinking more and more about doing the impossible.

Further Deterioration

Bernie was simply not taking his vitamins and supplements. He'd say he'd taken them, but they'd just sit there in their little dish on the drainboard. I could coax, argue, push, insist--but nothing would make him take them. He'd become suspicious of them, he wanted to know where they came from; he'd say he's saving them--nothing got them down his throat.

He was definitely getting more fragile, losing weight, although he ate well--it was like his metabolism was off. And he was beginning to walk with a stoop. Oh, I hated to see that, I just hated to see that. He'd always walked so ramrod straight. And his arms would hang at his sides, they didn't swing, just hang, like a zombie. Well, maybe it would have happened anyway, regardless of any pills.

He was getting slower and slower, more and more confused. He couldn't remember how to open and close the car door, or even where he was supposed to sit in the car. He was confused about how 'Sophie' got in the car and he couldn't find the inside door locks. Sometimes he tried to open the glove compartment to get out instead of his door. I had to always check his seatbelt. Either he forgot to hook it or he did it wrong.

He always seemed to have paper napkins or towels with him. He often kept a couple of them in his shirt pocket, and once he made neat little stacks of toilet paper squares on top of the closed toilet lid. And, of course, he frequently forgot to flush.

I had concerns about what trouble he might get into at night while I was trying to sleep, and he was frequently tucking the covers around me, then pulling them off my shoulders. When he hadn't been in the room for a while, I'd go looking for him and sometimes find him sound asleep standing, swaying in the middle of a room.

I never knew what I'd see in the morning: the clothes hamper was put into another room; the TV guide was neatly rolled and stuffed in his shoe; a cowboy figurine was moved to another spot; a throw rug from the hall was in the kitchen; the tissues and flashlight had been taken from the bedside table; several pairs of his clean socks were pushed into a small box; his shaver cord was wrapped around his toothbrush--he was really busy. I'd just put it all back and wait for the next go around. Once we went on errands and it was an hour or more before I noticed his toothbrush was sticking out of his shirt pocket. Don't ask--

Flying Notes

Being awake most of the night was really getting to me. So during the day, when Bernie was watching TV--or at least sitting there, dozing, I took the opportunity to nap myself. I was in Debby's old room with the door ajar so I could hear him, and he found me. He woke me with more tirades about men and breaking up the family. I asked him to just let me sleep.

He banged the door as he went out and in a short time a paper came flying in at me. What now? Papers came floating in every few minutes or so, until finally I got up and left the bed. But I saved the papers. Here are two of them. The mistakes are just as he made them, mistakes he'd have never made before.

Oh, God! My poor love, my poor love.

WHY ARE YOU HOSTILE AT ME. IVE DONE NOTHING TO DESERVE IT.	WHY ARE YOU SO HOSTILE AT ME IVE DONE NOTHING BUT LOVE AND CHARISH YOU, & I ALWAYS WILL PROTECT YOU

Doing My Best

I don't regret anything that I've done. I made the best decisions I could with the information that I had at the time. The fact that nothing panned out is just the way things went.

I'd most likely be beating myself up if I hadn't at least tried all that I did, but I won't beat myself for making the effort, even though there was scant success. Finally, I thought it's the end of the line, but if something new came along that looked promising, I'd still try it.

And there was one more odd thought. For all my talk of understanding Bernie's condition and knowing that there was no way to improve it, for all my fruitless research, planning and mental projections into the future, I still thought that things would go right again, that sooner or later, and I didn't know how, that Bernie and I would be the same again. Habit I guess. It just felt like what had always been would always be. Intellectually I knew that wasn't ever going to happen, but in my heart of hearts, that's what I believed.

"What'll I Do?"

Irving Berlin, 1923

Sometimes I thought I got too maudlin about all of this, although if I couldn't be maudlin with this, when could I? It's just that my nature is to be more buoyant. I kept floating back up to the surface like a balloon under water, and I thought that's the way it's going to be no matter what. But the words from that old song keep haunting me: "What'll I do?"

The idea of starting my life all over again, but alone, can be tremendously exhilarating and equally devastating. The big problem is that I'd had my life the way I wanted it. I had no great desire to travel more, to acquire new skills, or possessions. I've done more than most, and feel 'been there, done that, bought the T-shirt.' I've raised terrific children, established a comfortable nest, worked outside the home, and done far more than my share of volunteering. I wasn't opposed to just kicking back and taking it easy, especially after living always on the alert for several years, never knowing what might come next. After all, I was well into the *troisieme age* of life, just how much energy did I have left?

Then there was the question of companionship. Oh, sure, there were people in my life, but not a companion, not someone to sit quietly with, not someone with a common history, not anymore. So, I thought, 'what'll I do?'

Who would call me to the backyard to watch a flock of crows pecking the lawn? Who would point out the baby hatchlings hiding under the garage eaves, or the squirrel scampering up the telephone pole after eating an orange from the neighbor's tree? Who would show me the vibrant flower that sprang overnight from our ancient cactus, and tell me once again that we should take a picture of it?

And why did I so often say, "Honey, I'm busy right now," and not go look, thinking 'it's only a bird.' What was so important that it couldn't wait?

And who would ever again gently kiss and stroke my hands, telling me how soft and pretty they are? Who would offer me the last sip of his soda, the last bite of his pie? Who would share movie popcorn and let me hold the bag? Who would bring me my pink pillow and who would tease me about my always messy hair and tell me, no matter where we were, that I was the prettiest girl in the room? Who would ever again love me so completely without qualification? And who would ever again need me, to make him happy, and to smile?

◆TWELVE◆

June 1998

"Danger! Danger, Will Robinson!"

'Robot'
"Lost in Space" - 1965

I woke up alone with the sun, unsure of where Bernie was, so I went looking. He was roaming around the house. I found 'Sophie's dog dish on the sink with several prunes in it! I didn't know if he'd fed her anything or not--I was hoping not. There was also silverware, including another sharp knife left out, doors closed that I usually leave open, and things just out of place. I saw papers around my computer that had been moved and some diskettes from his old computer were nearby. Obviously he wasn't able to operate it, but it was one more thing to be concerned about.

But, surprise, surprise, his new razor, the one that had been missing for weeks, was on our dresser. When I asked him where he found it, he told me at the bowling alley. Well, why not? It had to have been someplace.

Some people think it's no big deal--taking care of someone who's just more forgetful than most, but it's not that way at all. Think of what it's like taking care of a fifteen-month-old toddler, knowing that you can't leave him unsupervised for a moment. You never know what he'll do. You can at least teach a toddler, correct him, explain something, and he'll learn, or even confine him for a while, but imagine, instead, a full grown adult in the same situation, only instead of progressing, he's getting worse and worse every day. Add to that, the person is still an adult, you really can't treat him like a baby, but you have to be on the alert every minute, clean up after him all the time, keep things out of his reach, lock dangerous things away. He doesn't sleep through the night and rarely sleeps during the day for any length of time. You don't get much rest. He's bigger and considerably stronger than you are, so you can't pick him up, send him to his room, put him to bed, or do much of anything to curb most of what he's doing.

Although the word had still never been spoken--except at UCLA where they didn't know and I'd been denying it--and even though he was never diagnosed with it no matter where I went, I knew all along that I was dealing with Alzheimer's. And except for possibly Aricept, which I had little faith in for Bernie, there wasn't anything to do for it anyway.

Still, outward denial had kept me afloat through some difficult times. I could have been wrong, but I knew I wasn't. Bernie's decline had been a textbook case. Except that he didn't wander, he did all the things an Alzheimer's patient does in the absolute order specified, and at about the same rate. If it continued this way, I could assume what was coming next. I had to see that he brushed his teeth and shaved, that he showered and got his clothes on correctly, that his shoes were laced and tied. It was only a matter of time until he might be unable to shower by himself, became incontinent. Maybe it wouldn't happen, but chances were that it would.

How would I be able to do it all alone with everything else that needed doing? I couldn't ignore the fact that I was pushing 70, no matter how strong I continued to feel. And I wasn't getting any younger, that's for sure. It was hard enough when a full-time caregiver was young and had some professional training, but I had neither youth nor training, and I didn't think I'd be able to do all that was going to be necessary for years to come, even if I got respite.

Certainly I could get people in the house, but I knew Bernie would not like that and I wouldn't like it either. We'd be stumbling all over each other, angry and annoyed most of the time. Besides, it wouldn't stop the dangerous behavior; it'd just be placing one more person in harm's way, putting off the inevitable. It was an option, but not the best one. I knew what I had to do, and I knew I had the strength to do it, but it was so hard, I just couldn't let go, not yet, not yet, I just couldn't let go of him.

My Precious Scarecrow

Sometimes Bernie was very lucid, he realized that his mind was going and he would say something about his brain. He'd tell me how he'd have to look into a way to fix it. After all, he'd always fixed everything that needed fixing, everything from cars to clocks. It used to astonish me. It seemed he only had to look at something and, like magic, it would work again.

Now he was like the Scarecrow on his way to Oz. He had heart and courage to spare, perfect in so many ways, 'if he only had a brain.' I'd written enough about the inane things he did all day long--and most of the night as well. He couldn't even complete a rational sentence most of the time, and he knew it. His lips quivered, the words tumbled and jumbled, and I'd just say 'yes.' I'd tell anyone else around to agree with the sounds, the words wouldn't make sense. Any form of 'yes, I think so' or 'you're right,' would do to make him think that he had communicated something. Don't ask him to explain what he meant; he wouldn't be able to do it.

So I lived with this lovable scarecrow that looked and sounded just like my handsome husband. But he didn't move like him, didn't talk like him, didn't act like him at all. He was like a robot on auto-pilot, going through programmed motions, but not having any sense of what he was doing, much less why. And so, very late one night, I telephoned Matt.

It's Time

All I said was, "Do you think it's time?" And he said 'yes.' There was no need for any further explanation between us, although we did briefly review Bernie's condition, all our futures, other options, but we both knew it was time.

Matt immediately began to take over; shifting a burden from me that I didn't know was so heavy until it was being lifted. From the list of facilities I'd already made, we settled on Royale Park in Pasadena, about forty minutes away. It was near another of our HMO offices so we could have his medical records transferred there from the one close to our house.

As soon as the arrangements were made, Matt began to talk to me about all I'd done for Bernie, the things I'd tried, the places I'd taken him, my strength, my love, my honoring my commitment, doing the right thing. I wish I'd known he was going to say all of that, I'd have taped it! The truth is, he had done the same, offering me his strength, giving both of us his love, honoring his father, also doing the right thing, not only as a son, but as a decent human being. Neither one of us could have done it any other way.

So there was one of those silver linings that sometimes come with tragedy, a little epiphany that you knew was there anyway, but now came shining through like a sudden rainbow between showers.

The hardest part was yet to come.

Doing the Impossible

It had become impossible. Nothing would make him sleep unless I was in bed with him and then it was only for a short time. I had to be in the same room with him every minute, could not be out of his sight. I could sit with him in the den and do my embroidery, crossword puzzles, watch TV or read--but that was it. I couldn't go anywhere that he didn't follow me. We couldn't go for a walk because he was too slow and stooped over. I couldn't go by myself because I couldn't leave him alone. It was so bad that when I went to the bathroom, he'd knock on the door wanting to know if there was anything he could do to help! I was so exhausted that half the time I didn't know what I was doing and half the time I was all mixed up. I knew I was at the end of my rope, barely holding on. If I continued like this, I'd end up in an institution myself. I'd begun to count the days until we can get him into Royale--the days, the minutes, the mini-seconds.

How do you do that? How do you lock away the one constant in your life since childhood? Don't ask me. I don't know. But Karley knew. She was the Director at Royale, our primary contact, the one who showed us around, the one who would guide us through the impossible. Matt and I had taken Bernie out to Royale for lunch the week before. Karley ate with us and it was all very congenial. Bernie agreed it was a nice place. There was no talk about his staying there, just an afternoon lunch in a pleasant restaurant.

"D-N-R"

I couldn't just walk in the door, hand him off and say, "Here's a new resident." I had to get a TB test, medical forms filled out from the psychiatrist and his primary physician, things like that. When I called the two doctors, the first thing each one said to me was, "You're doing the right thing." As deeply as it hurt, I knew it was the right thing--the *only* thing. Still, their telling me without my asking was appreciated.

There was one other critically important document I had to give to Royale--Bernie's Living Will. We had each signed a lot of legal papers about six years ago. As I recall, we signed in an almost cavalier manner--of course, neither one of us wanted to needlessly suffer, what fool would? We both agreed if we were terminal, we didn't want any heoric medical efforts made. At that time, Bernie was quite lucid. I'm sure neither one of us thought much about the reality of our being in a position to actually have to make such a decision, and certainly not so soon.

But, now, here it was. Bernie was in good health, I didn't expect anything to happen because of the Alzheimer's, but he could have a heart attack, a bad accident, one never knows. Maybe I wouldn't be available at such a critical moment, so I felt it was only reasonable to give Royale guidance in Bernie's wishes.

I handed Karley the papers and she said that they'd mark his file: "D-N-R." D-N-R? I didn't know what that meant. "Do Not Resuscitate," she told me. Ah, I understood, and I was grateful we had signed those documents. I didn't feel any additional burden, at least not at that moment, about if and when the time came. The decision had already been made for me.

The truth is, I felt that Bernie had suffered so much, been through such torture, hell and damnation, that he shouldn't have to go through any more of it needlessly. He deserved his peace.

Our Life

Matt announced early on that he and Zeli, his friend from Brazil, were going to take care of arranging everything in Bernie's room. I couldn't have been given a better gift. I'd been dreading the task. Zeli had been in our lives for about a year, and although she didn't know Bernie before his dementia, she'd been very kind and thoughtful toward him.

Finally the day came for Bernie's placement and we went out to Royale to have lunch again. I was so roiled up, I didn't know how I was going to get through it. At one point, Bernie said, "I don't belong here," but nobody responded. Then Karley asked him if he'd like to join in one of the group activities. He got up, followed her and never looked back at us.

While Bernie was gone, I went alone to his room to see what Matt and Zeli had done. I stood there slowly turning round and round, looking at my life. A wicker love seat, just like the one from our bedroom was there, with a new floral cushion. Bernie's clothes were neatly hung and carefully placed in drawers. There were pictures of Debby and Jean-François, their boys, our house with the roses out front, Matt and Bernie with our race cars, and racing trophies on the bureau. In the closet was the little yellow Formica table Bernie made when I was pregnant with Debby, and on that were some of Bernie's tools in a small red tool chest.

Over the closet was the sign from his first business: "Weiss Engineering Co." and on the shelf above were a dozen of the old analog meters from the collection he'd been assembling for years.

There were racing magazines and engineering books on the table and technical charts on the walls. In his wallet, Bernie always carried a picture of the roadster he courted me in and a photo of me alone on our wedding day. Now, they were framed on the wall, too. But the other snapshot he always carried, the one of me in a bathing suit at Venice Beach, the one I'd sent to him in Korea, had disappeared.

So there I stood alone, crying silently, looking at my life When Karley came in, she told me that she'd never seen a room done with more love--and that Bernie had gone off on a bus with the other residents to a museum. He never thought to say good-bye.

It's Over

Matt and I came home and sat in the den, silent for the most part. Until that moment, I hadn't noticed how hard the impact of the loss of his father had been on him. They had been so close, but now he was letting me see it a little, and the reality of it was in the room with us. I'd been too consumed with my own sorrow to notice his before. I felt bad about that, for him and Debby, the grandsons, it was such a loss for all of us. After a while he went home and I was finally, fully, and irrevocably, alone.

We had agreed that we wouldn't tell anyone about placing Bernie in a home until after he was settled in. I didn't want to be answering questions, getting advice, or explaining anything. Now I had to tell his siblings, and mine as well. I made the calls, voice choking, eyes filling, as brief as possible. With that, the news would eventually spread through both extended families. I kept assuring them that I was OK, that I'd *be* OK. I was still strong--you had to be strong to do what I'd just done. The catch in my voice was only momentary. I knew it made things sound worse to them than they actually were.

Because of the time difference, I had to wait until late night to call Debby, who already knew of our plans, but everyone and everything else could wait. She was coming to visit in a few weeks. I was anxious to see her, to have something to look forward to. After we hung up, 'Sophie' curled up in her bed, and I crawled alone into mine.

◆THIRTEEN◆

June 1998

"Life is what happens to you while you're busy making other plans."

John Lennon

I woke early the next morning, surprised that I'd slept soundly through the night for the first time in years. With an overwhelming sense of freedom, I could literally see my physical, emotional, and mental burdens lifting from me and floating off like the bright hot air balloons that fill an Albuquerque sky.

What was this? This couldn't be normal? My life's companion for fifty years, my sweet love, and sometimes my most annoying aggravation, my rock, my stabilizer, my emotional repository wasn't here and I was feeling--dare I say it?--I was feeling happy!

Why didn't I miss him? Where were all the tears for someone I loved and married because he was the one person I wanted to be with all the time, the one who made me feel pretty, safe and always comfortable? Once, when we were very young, I told him that when I was with him, I had a mental picture of a cat curled up sleeping in front of a burning hearth, a man in a nearby rocker smoking a pipe. He said that sounded like pure contentment to him, and so, I guess it was.

It didn't take long to figure it out though. I was happy because I was so relieved to have shed the responsibilities of caregiving; it wasn't because Bernie was gone. I didn't miss him now because in truth, little by little, without either one of us realizing it, I'd already been without him for a long, long time.

I couldn't remember the last time I'd had anything like a normal conversation with him. I'd grown used to agreeing with anything that came out of his mouth, not really listening or trying to understand. Asking him why he did something just resulted in some sort of nonsensical response. But I kept up the pretense.

Watching TV or going to the movies with him didn't produce any reasonable comments. Mostly he forgot what he saw as it was happening, or else came up with a completely inappropriate response. He basically stopped reading menus in restaurants, usually saying he'd have the same thing I had ordered. He even stopped advising me how to drive--and that was a change, believe me.

I lied to him all the time just to avoid explanations, confrontations, or the truth, none of which he'd understand, or even worse, would only frighten him more. It didn't matter that I lied, because he'd forget what I said almost instantly and then never remember if I said something different later. It wasn't like I had to keep my stories straight and it certainly wasn't that I wanted to deceive him. I'd have given anything to be able to be honest with him, but I wouldn't be able to function if that's what I had to do.

Subconsciously I had probably been distancing myself for a long time. I knew what was coming and if I hadn't started to protect myself, as well as Bernie, I'd have turned into mush, and that wouldn't have helped either one of us. And I did have this need to protect us both, I just hadn't been all that aware of it.

In fact, I thought I'd been doing quite well. If it hadn't been that Bernie began night walking, keeping me endlessly awake, raging about other men, and a fear that he might hit me, I would have continued on in the same vein.

He Did Everything Right

That's what hurt the most. He did everything right.

The day was still young when I had the mother of all crying jags, yelling, screaming to the empty bedroom, "he did everything right." He tried so hard, he sacrificed so much, he gave so much, and now this! It wasn't fair, it just wasn't fair. He deserved better than this, he'd earned it, he was entitled, he was just damned entitled!

I knew it was natural to idealize Bernie at that moment, to accentuate the positive and eliminate the negative. But if Bernie hadn't had more good in him than not, I'd have never stayed around so long. Yes, I was certainly furious with him many times, but I could never intentionally hurt him anymore than I could kick a puppy for chewing my slipper. He worked so hard and so long. He was so faithful, so loyal, so reliable. He never missed a Little League game or a school function. He was the one who pasted blue sparkles on the hooves of Debby's horse when she was in parades, for goodness sake. What kind of payback was this? So he wasn't perfect, so he could be a chauvinist (always in denial, to be sure), but never cruel, never oppressive, never demanding.

And, frequently, he could easily be engrossed in his own thoughts so that sometimes I had to really work hard to get his attention, although now I think it was possibly the beginnings of this horrible disease. And he could make me so angry at times I just wanted to smash him and then soon loved him and couldn't remember why I was upset.

I was chastising myself for the times I'd pushed him away, turned out of the room, didn't answer, didn't explain. How could I have done those things to him? And I knew I didn't tell him enough times how much I appreciated him and all that he did for me and the children.

The crying and accusing the air went on until I was wholly exhausted, or did you think that because I was no longer his sole caregiver, I was going to live alone happily ever after? Fat chance. I thought of how much he was going to miss our family life, which meant everything to him. I thought of how comfortable we were because of how hard he worked, and how smart and generous he always was, and what did he get to enjoy for it? I'll tell you what, *bubpkis*, that's what. Life sucked. It truly sucked.

"When All is Said and Done"

All is never all said and all is never all done. Oh, you know, the ripple effect, whatever one says and does affects everyone else, down the block, down the ages, six degrees of separation and all that. There's always something more, everyone's life is a series of events melding one into the other.

But I had to plunk down a period in my life NOW, like I would at the end of a sentence chiseled in stone. It didn't mean that I didn't go back and re-read that sentence, but it did mean I recognized that it couldn't be changed--much as I might have wanted to rewrite it, I couldn't, anymore than I could hold back the sunrise. I might read it again and again, to cry or laugh, but I couldn't change it, and besides, the next sentence was already being carved, whether I wanted it to be or not.

I had this dreadful feeling that Bernie was being left behind, and surrounded by 150 patients and staff every day, he was more alone than I was. He should have been in his home, our beautiful home, where I could hold him close and we could be together like we were always meant to be. He deserved no less, and I didn't deserve this wounded heart.

But the period was set HERE and I couldn't change it. So when certain pictures made me cry, I didn't keep looking at them. When old melodies made me sad, I stopped listening. His clothes, his tools, his car--and then there were his car keys--keys that he'd never use again--keys that still hung on a hook next to the back door--his keys where he left them for the last time--still hanging there.

I didn't know what would come next, but I knew that whatever it might be, I'd have to go with it. I learned very young that I couldn't stop the unhappy tides of fate that came along, but I could float. As soon as one wave passed, it was only a matter of time until another wave came along, so in the meantime, I might just as well float. Worse things could happen. But, at least for the moment, I was floating.

Adjusting

I visited Bernie once or twice a week. I would call him and sometimes he had the switchboard call me. On the phone he asked me to come and get him, and I said I would to placate him, but I couldn't bring him home, and that hurt, to know he'd never be home again.

The staff said that he asked for me all the time at first, but eventually less as time went on. He seemed to be making contact with the other patients. He kissed the cheeks of the women and slapped the backs of the men, 'hail fellow, well met' stuff. They said that he participated in the activities, even sang and danced! But I didn't see how the patients could communicate with each other. It was all just babble to my ears.

The staff picked him up at night on the TV monitors when he left his room and walked the halls. They'd ask if he wanted a banana, or needed to use the bathroom, then put him back to bed. In no time, he'd be up again.

A few times he'd be awake and aware when I would visit, but because he didn't sleep at night, or because of the meds they gave him to sleep, he often just kept nodding off and I sat there like a dolt. After a while, I'd go home. When he woke up, he probably thought my visit was a dream. Who knows?

The Girlfriend

One woman set her cap for Bernie as soon as he came in the door. Born in Scotland, called 'Scottie,' she wouldn't leave him alone. Well, I could hardly fault her taste in men.

When I sat next to him in the lounge, she'd come by and pat his shoulders in a very proprietary fashion. Hannah, one of the staff, would come over and lead her away, telling her to leave Bernie alone, that I was his wife. But she came back again and again. She talked to me, explaining something, babbling, and it was impossible to understand her. Like Bernie, her words just didn't compute.

They told me that she banged on the door to his room, wanting to get inside, and when told, 'he's married,' she'd get angry and say 'no, he's mine.' Once she tried to pull him away from my arm. At first, I didn't believe Bernie wholly reciprocated her feelings. I'd seen him relate to other women there, he kind of spread his attention around.

As time went on though, Hannah told me that the two of them often walked together, holding hands, and sometimes kissed--but he called her 'Betty.' I didn't think he was able to tell anyone what her name was--to him, she was 'Betty.' It was more than a little strange because she didn't look any more like me than Abbott looked like Costello, but if she was 'Betty' to him, then so be it.

Since this had been going on, he hadn't asked to phone me either, so something was happening. I knew that the time might come when he wouldn't remember me at all, maybe this was the start of it, and it wouldn't be easy.

People asked me how I could possibly stand to see him do this, but I was happy for him. I didn't think that the man who walked with Scottie was really my husband--he was a human shell who looked the same, with the same name, but who would never do such a thing if he weren't demented.

It might sound false, but I was glad. She gave him individual attention, comfort and affection--things that I couldn't give him when I wasn't there and things the staff didn't have time to give. I knew such behavior was common practice among people like this, and nothing more was going to happen between them, I was sure of that--well, pretty sure.

Between Bernie and me, I was the one set adrift. He was surrounded by people, cared for and looked after. But except for 'Sophie,' I was alone. No one was fussing over me, doing for me. He was drifting away from me, but I couldn't drift away from him because I had normal awareness. I don't mean to complain, I was just thinking of the irony.

Family Visits

Debby and her family came for the summer, and we'd all go out to visit Bernie--Debby, Jean-François, me and the boys. But he couldn't 'see' Guillaume and Justin just inches from his nose. His eyes, unclear, looked down or out across the room past their faces. I tried to move his head, to make him see them, but he couldn't. He was unable to recognize his own picture or read his name on the door to his room. It was an incredible phenomenon. I asked him to look at us in a wall mirror, but he wouldn't. I don't think he liked mirrors.

He didn't hear me either. I could stand behind him, touch his back, talk directly into his ear, and he didn't turn or acknowledge me in any way, and he no longer responded to my nuzzling him. In just a few weeks, he stopped telling me that he loved me and that I was so beautiful--and I missed it. What a bummer. I expected some of this might happen, but not that he couldn't see or hear us.

July 4th, 1998

Debby and I, Debby's friend and her mom, whose husband had been in a fetal position for seven years with Alzheimer's, had gone to UCLA for a show at Royce Hall. What a foursome! Guess what the two moms talked about? Ah, well.

During intermission, a young man, early 20's, made his way through the crowd to talk to me. I was trying to remember who he was, when I realized that he was a complete stranger. But he told me about his mother, about the time they saw 'Cats' here, and 'Hello, Dolly,' and how good the shows were. He wanted to talk and I let him. It was obvious he was retarded. His mother waited in the aisle for us to finish our conversation and then they walked off.

I told Debby, my beautiful, healthy, normal daughter, that I really didn't have that much to feel sad about. She understood, at least Dad had had his life.

Hundreds of people were in that auditorium. Why did he seek me out instead of someone else? How do these moments of fate happen? I know there are worse things in life than Alzheimer's--but Alzheimer's still hurts--it really, really, really hurts.

Fireworks

Later, as usual, we went to watch fireworks. I couldn't remember how long we'd been doing this--well over 40 years, but it was the first time for Guillaume and Justin. I thought Debby wanted them to experience something from her childhood and this was fun. I'm sure they liked it, but I could only think about Bernie's not being with us, about his not seeing his grandsons enjoy the spectacle. I knew he wasn't even thinking about us or the Fourth of July. My healthy, vibrant, brilliant, handsome, strong man, who so loved his family and these gatherings was lying in a bed alone, his mind slipping silently away, while in the darkness fireworks lit up the night, ear-shattering booms filled the sky and everyone else just 'ooh-d' and 'ahh-d' away.

•FOURTEEN•

August 1998

Nice People

On our next family visit, Bernie had several small scabs on his right elbow and knee. They didn't look like abuse injuries and I wasn't surprised, having been told that he fell and that they found him on the floor more than once. Scottie came by and easily led him away from our little family. I don't think he realized anymore how we fit into his life. We were nice people who came to see him, but he didn't care anymore if we came or not, he was bonding with the others.

The Punching-Bag Clown

You know those balloon-clown toys that kids knock down only to have them pop up again and again? Well, that's how I was feeling. As soon as I stood up, I got knocked down again, and it was the pits--it was the pit of the pits.

I had an appointment to take him to the new doctor at our HMO. I'd thought he was adjusting well at Royale and felt pretty good about things until I walked in the front door--they were waiting for me. In Karley's office I was told things I could hardly believe. How could she say such outlandish things?

Bernie was getting more and more aggressive. He broke a lamp and chased a nurse down the hall with it! He was yelling that 'they' were trying to kill him, and when attendants called Karley to try to calm him down, he warned her to be careful, that 'they' were trying to kill her, too. Oh, God, that was real paranoia. He still didn't sleep at night, and they wanted me to tell the doctor that he should be hospitalized until medications could stabilize him!

Oh, great, just great! They thought that Dano, his assigned nurse, should go with me to the doctor's office and I was more than happy to have him. I didn't know what Bernie might do. What a mess.

I told the new doctor what Royale wanted, but he didn't hospitalize him. Instead he prescribed a different drug. Within days Royale said it made him less aggressive and more easily directed. I thought things were going along pretty well for a bit, and on my next visit he hugged me, tight, as if he was really glad to see me, and I was pleased. After an hour or so, I was ready to leave.

Well, punch me, punch me, punch me! At the front desk I was ambushed again by staff. Did you think I could get away that easily? I had to take him back to the doctor and these were the things they wanted me to tell him:

He paces all the time.

He tries to leave the facility.

He was getting aggressive again. He got right in people's faces, showing real anger.

It took two or three people to control him.

He was up at night, again.

They wanted to increase the dosage for the medicine.

We stood at the front desk discussing all of this, and Bernie joined in the conversation. He didn't have any idea we were talking about him, he thought it was someone else.

And--and this was a BIG 'AND'--he and Scottie were escalating their relationship. Hannah was reluctant to tell me some of the things they were doing, but I pushed her for it. Scottie sits on his lap and there's a lot of touching. She wants to spend the night with him, and maybe he felt the same way. They were getting harder and harder to separate, she'd get very angry when they'd tell her about me and didn't want to hear it. Wouldn't you think I'd feel some jealousy? But I didn't. I just felt, I don't know--numb--I guess. Part of me felt OK and part of me felt repulsed.

When I finally left, Bernie turned really angry. No doubt he thought I was going out to meet another lover. Well, what's good for the goose is good for the gander, and all such stuff. He'd probably be harder for the staff to handle now--but I didn't care. I was going home to collapse. Soon there'd be another doctor's appointment for me to take him to.

"I'm Doing Just Fine."

That's what I always told people, I'm doing just fine. "I'm OK, really I am, I'm OK," because what else could I say?

On one level I really was OK. I didn't think I'd have any sort of collapse, and I planned to build a new life for myself. I'd be OK if I didn't get hit by a truck, I was confident of that.

As soon as Deb went back to France, I had plans for some activities. Good grief, if you can't find things to do and people to meet in Los Angeles then you must be six feet under.

I still had a lot of my good life anyway. Besides my responsibilities toward Bernie and his care, I had my children and grandchildren, sisters, in-laws, neighbors, a friend or two, and 'Sophie,' of course. I wasn't exactly alone. And my home was important to me, there was always something needed doing, and I was comfortable there. So, I was doing OK--except--except--

Where was the child who loved me in grammar school, the boy who took me to my senior prom, who courted me, the man I married, the father of my children, the one who made me financially independent, who nursed me whenever I was sick, who loved, protected, and cared for me with all his body and heart, the one who was going to grow old with me--the one who wasn't there anymore? Yeah, I was OK, who wouldn't be?

A Morning Wake-Up

The phone rang before 7:30 a.m. It was the night nurse from Royale. She said she knew I was coming in to take Bernie to the doctor and she wanted to prepare me--(heart skips a beat)--for when I see him--(another skip).

When she checked on him last night, his face was scraped on his forehead and the bridge of his nose. She didn't know how he had done it, it looked like carpet burns. When she asked him, he said he was doing his exercises for his track and field. (Heartbeat slows.) Was he facedown on the carpet? She doesn't know, but the mental picture disturbs me (heart is waiting).

What else? I knew there was a 'what else' in her voice. And then she told me; and it also explained why Hannah had handed me a pair of his freshly laundered shorts the day before. He'd lost bowel control, had soiled in the hallway, and they thought he did that on purpose because they wouldn't let him do something--but Bernie's never been vindictive, and certainly not like that! But, then, Bernie had been doing a lot of things he'd never done before.

And he had messed a couple of times on his bathroom floor, like he'd gone in there, but forgot to sit on the toilet. And if that wasn't bad enough, he'd smeared it on the wall! Well, I thought I was going to die, I just knew I was going to die. And I knew Bernie would die, too, if he had any idea he had done this. And he'd probably kill me, anyway, if he knew I would be writing about it. But I had decided to record everything, that it was important to do so--(although I've held a few things back that are too painful to write about--but it's 99 percent complete)--I just didn't think there was going to be so much (you should pardon the expression), so much crap!

Oh, yes, of course, there was more. Sometimes they'd find Bernie roaming buck naked in the hallways! I was told it wasn't all that uncommon with Alzheimer's, but it didn't make me feel a whole lot better. Good grief! Naked! Bernie! No way!

And he'd hit some of the staff, hard, so hard that it hurt. I wasn't surprised that it hurt, he had incredible strength. It pleased me to know he still had that inborn strength, but I'll bet the staff wasn't pleased when he hit them.

And in spite of his eating well, he was still losing weight. I could only think again that his metabolism was somehow shutting down. I was sure I weighed much more than he did now--and that really frosted me.

All this had been very distressing. (Heart was still beating--barely--it had taken so many hits, it needed time to recoup.) In a while I dragged myself from bed, fed 'Sophie,' gulped coffee, whatever, and headed for the freeways. The doctor would be waiting and I'd have all that to add to the list.

It turned out that placing Bernie in a care facility did not really relieve me of my caregiving responsibilities. I simply could not get out from under.

Displaying All the Symptoms

Bernie was nothing if not thorough, and he was that way now with this disease. So far he had displayed all the symptoms I'd heard and read about--he'd only left out wandering. And I knew that there would be more to come. I couldn't have handled all of this at home, I just couldn't, and it was only going to get worse.

When I saw him, his face was a mess. It did look like carpet burns, except there was also a gouge-like wound on his nose, like he had fallen against something. There was no way to know what happened. Dano went with us to the doctor again.

The doctor increased his medication, but wanted him to start seeing a psychiatrist. Bernie's condition was now beyond his general practice. I had learned that all of Bernie's actions: forgetting that we were married, raging at me, never closing doors, getting dressed in the middle of the night, not sleeping--all of it was normal Alzheimer's behavior. How in the name of heaven did people live through this? With nothing left to say to the doctor, we went back to Royale.

As soon as we got inside the door, Scottie was at Bernie. She examined his nose and forehead, concerned, telling him, in her babble, how to care for it, asking my opinion. I didn't know what she said, it didn't make any sense to me, but I said 'yes' anyway. With everything else, why did I have to be nice to that woman? But I didn't want to offend her, to hurt her, or worse yet, to get her riled up--but still...

When I was leaving, Bernie's bottom lip was quivering, tears forming. I couldn't bear to see his face, the face I loved so much, once so rugged now crumpled like a frightened child's, and I knew, in spite of Scottie, he wanted to come home with me--and God knows, I wanted that, too, more than anything, I wanted that, too. My heart and soul were exhausted from leaving him, seeing his fear, his loneliness, being abandoned alone without me. I rushed blindly out the front door, the receptionist yelling after me, "Betty, slow down!" But I kept running to the car, crying, and hurried home ASAP, telling myself the whole way, 'watch your driving, dummy.'

Punch the clown, punch the clown, punch the clown!

A Special Visitor

From time to time, I took 'Sophie' with me to Royale. When I took her inside the lobby, a small knot of patients would form around, petting and hugging her, blabbering something or other, enjoying the moment. But not Bernie. He didn't 'see' her. I'd bring her over to his chair, pulling his hand, forcing it onto her back, willing him to pet her, to respond, but he never did.

'Sophie,' being a cool cat for a dog tolerated everything they did, but not terribly well. Too many hands, walkers, smells, and nattering voices made her edgy. Since it wasn't helping Bernie, I stopped bringing her. She didn't object.

Adjustment Difficulties

Debby and her family were going to return to France in a few days. I loved them all, and the boys were so cute, such a joy, it was impossible to keep from pinching and hugging them. When we visited Bernie, Jean-François talked with him about computers and such--as much as Bernie could 'talk.' I thought that was good for Bernie. He always interacted well with other men.

But he was not adjusting as well as we had hoped. Even with his meds, now raised to three times a day, he still got aggressive with other patients, hit them, and talked about suicide. If I'd thought aggression was not like him, I can say that suicide was even less so. He wasn't the sort to give up--ever--about anything. He was a true Aries, the ram. He'd see something, a goal, and he went to it. Nothing stood in his way. But now he had just enough reasoning power left to know what his life was like, that Royale was not a life for him, that in spite of good care, he was a prisoner.

Maybe my visits--our family visits--were holding back his adjusting. He'd only been at Royale for two months.

We'll Always Have Sunday

I am writing about Sunday now because Monday was a nightmare--it wasn't over yet. So, here goes--Sunday.

We all went out to see Bernie--Debby and her gang, Matt, Zeli, and me. We found him with Scottie, but Hannah quickly took her away. Sitting around, we had a nice chat. Bernie let me hold his hand, he gave me his sappy 'I love you so much' look, and participated as much as possible. He did talk about sealed boxes in the garage just outside his room, none of it making any sense, but that was OK, we all knew that he was often off in another realm.

I noticed that he was wearing a new electronic monitor on his wrist. He and Scottie had actually gotten out together. It's the third one they've put on him. Somehow he was able to get the first two off. I was glad to see it replaced, it made me feel a little less anxious.

His face had healed, all the bruises and scabs were gone, so we took some photos. The day was good, except that I had a hard time keeping my composure when everyone said their individual 'goodbyes' because I knew that if Debby came back next summer, he would probably be a lot worse, and I thought she understood that, too. I could tell by her eyes and the way she hugged me--tight. No matter how good things seemed now, he was never going to get any better--that was a given we all understood. It could be the last time we would all be together like this, our little family, or anyway, the last time Bernie would be so aware of us all.

On the ride home, we talked about how well the medicine was finally working. How 'with it' Bernie seemed, how calm, easygoing, and participating. We all agreed that it had been a great Sunday, a perfect sendoff for Deb and her family to go back to France the next day.

◆FIFTEEN◆

August 1998

An Unbelievable Nightmare

Who dreams up these horrors? Short of dying, was there never going to be an end to Bernie's being jerked around like this? What in God's name did this most decent, loving, generous, gentle man ever do to deserve such torture? And don't give me any half-baked philosophies about mysterious plans and bad things happening to good people. If it makes you feel good--go for it, feel good, but as for me--it doesn't help one whit. It isn't that I think for a moment that I feel any better or worse than anyone else going through this miserable morass, it's just that sometimes things happen, no matter what one does or believes, and all I could do was learn to live with it. Not everything has to have an explanation.

It was watching Bernie, being unable to even offer very much comfort that tore at me. It made even less sense to think that he'd be getting some wondrous heavenly reward, some sort of afterlife brownie points for all the pain he was being forced to endure, or that it was bad karma from his previous lives. Gimme a break. Nothing was worth the price he was paying.

Now there was another early morning phone call from Royale. For some time they'd been telling me about his violence, hitting other patients, chasing staff, but he always calmed down. This time, he went too far.

It started in the dining room with his biting other patients and twisting their arms. This was astonishing; I wouldn't think that Bernie even knew how to twist someone's arm. Then he ran to the lounge, began to throw chairs, kicked a table, and tossed a birdcage across the room--yes, with the bird still in it! He had to be in such pain to do this, to try to slice through his mental torment, to smash anything and anyone in his way in a futile attempt to escape this incessant madness.

The police were called, it took several to subdue him, then he was taken to a hospital. Great, just great. I was being told, in effect, that they could not keep him at Royale unless he was stabilized. Of course, of course, I understood that. But what would I do, where could he go? I was told to wait, someone would contact me.

Soon I got a call from the hospital. Bernie was handcuffed to a bed. Otherwise, he was just fine for the moment, having a casual chat with the police. He hadn't been hurt, had calmed down all on his own, but had no memory of what he had done, and no memory of ever living at Royale. Going in and out between violence and calm, he would be transferred to our HMO hospital. Because he was in the process of being moved again, I stayed home to wait for another phone call to tell me where he'd be.

Finally it came. After some discussion, the doctor said that she was committing him involuntarily to our HMO's lockdown mental institution in Downtown Los

Angeles where he could be restrained and stabilized. Honestly, I wasn't sure what she said--I just blurted out, "You're doing what?"

Read these words, words that have never been in my personal life before with these meanings, and with such an in-your-face intensity until now:

COMMITTED	INVOLUNTARY	MENTAL HEALTH
LOCKDOWN	RESTRAINED	HANDCUFFED
STABILIZE	PSYCHIATRIC	EVALUATED

Handcuffed, involuntary commitment, lockdown--the words were slamming into me with such force I could barely breathe.

By now I thought he'd be terrified, and I wanted to see him, to help soothe his fears, give him someone to hold on to, but the doctor said 'no,' not yet. She thought in his present state, he'd just push me away anyway. "You don't want to see this," she told me. "Let us handle it, spare yourself." I didn't want to 'spare myself,' I wanted to be with him, but I didn't know where he was or how long he'd be there. I scoured all the information I had about our HMO and could not find anything about a lockdown mental institution. I had to trust, I had to wait.

I had already visualized his wild rampage at Royale, his face contorted, throwing things, attacking people, kicking, the bird flung through the air, seeing uniformed police rush through the door, wrestling him down, handcuffed to a bed--he'd never been handcuffed in his life, never. It was all pretty hard to get into my head--that all of this was really happening to Bernie. Not my sweet Bernie, how could it be?

And this all gave me time to reflect on things I had done, decisions I'd made, doing what seemed best, hoping for the best. More than ever, I realized I'd done the right thing placing him even though that's not what I ever planned to do, never really wanted to do, but how is a grandmother like me, alone, expected to control and care for a grown man when it took a professional staff and police officers to subdue him. Anything could have happened to either one of us--to a stranger for all I knew. As much as it hurt, I knew I hadn't made the decision any too soon.

Now it was all out of my hands. I had to believe these people, that they would care for Bernie with skill and compassion. There was no other option. I didn't know any of them, didn't even know for certain where they all were, just voices on the telephone. He was being handed off like a hot potato from one place to another. I appreciated their calling, keeping me informed, telling me who they were, the name of the facilities, but I was on the other side of town and wasn't sure where to find him--I just had to trust them. They had always taken good care of us, I had few complaints and nothing major--I had to trust.

Deb and her family had gone back to France that morning, I was alone. It had been a day full of phone calls and troubled concerns. Mercifully it finally ended. I told 'Sophie' to go to bed. Tomorrow someone would call me from someplace and it would start all over again.

Lockdown

A doctor called me from lockdown! The very word made me cringe. The clank of doors, the jangle of keys, white uniforms. Oh, make no mistake, it was a prison. But, at least, I finally knew where he was.

He said Bernie had asked him personally to call me. He wanted to know Bernie's medical history, and told me what meds he would be given. It sounded like a lot to me.

Bernie was on a 72-hour hold. The doctor asked what I wanted the outcome to be, and I told him I hoped Bernie could be stabilized and returned to Royale, that I had spoken to them about that, and they were in accord. He said he thought they could do that, but he might have to apply to the Court for an additional 14-day hold until they got the meds right. After that, if he was still not stabilized, there would have to be a hearing. There'd be a referee, and a social worker to act as Bernie's advocate, doctors and other people, but, if it came to it, he didn't think further confinement would be denied.

He also asked me if I had conservatorship, if I agreed to his treatment, and could he call Royale. I told him that I have all the authority, all the necessary papers, that Bernie and I signed them while he was still quite lucid, when everyone was telling me that there was nothing wrong with him, that he was perfectly normal. It had all been done legally, consulting with doctors and attorneys, and of course he had my permission to treat him. Where else could I take him? I'd already tried everything I could think of, and I knew this doctor wasn't going to make him well. There would be no miracle workers for Bernie. Maybe the prayers people told me that they'd offered along the way had helped, but any such divine intervention wasn't working now.

Visiting hours were only from 7:00 p.m. to 8:00 p.m., but the doctor said he would leave instructions at the gate for me to come in the afternoon, so that's what I decided to do. If Bernie had asked for me to be called, he must want to see me, and I had to see him.

"Don't Give Up On Me"

The facility was surrounded by steel rod fencing with curved spikes on top--to keep people in or out? The parking entrance had a heavy metal gate and a nearby intercom that I was told to speak into. I explained that I had permission to visit my husband. The 'voice' held a conference with someone inside, the gate opened by itself then clanged closed behind me. I did as I was instructed and followed a blue line to Security.

Inside the lobby I signed the register and was directed to an elevator where someone would meet me. I could hear my name being announced over a walkie-talkie, telling Security I was coming. A guard opened the elevator with a key and we went up to the 'Elopement Area.' Elopement? To leave without permission? Passing through a locked door, I saw an old man shuffling across the hall with an attendant guiding him, and my whole body lurched when I realized the 'old man' was my Bernie.

He was wearing slipper-socks and blue hospital 'scrubs' with food stains on the front. His eyes were red-rimmed, he looked thinner, and his chin was resting on his chest. He hadn't been shaved and his hair was lank. I couldn't get him to raise his head, so I stooped in front of him, turning up my face so he could see it, talking to him, trying to get a response. We sat down at a table and I kept thinking he was overmedicated, that his head was drooping forward even more because of it. He looked like other patients at Royale who sat dozing in lounge chairs all day, and I desperately didn't want that for him. I wanted him to lift his head, but he couldn't seem to, maybe he didn't even try.

The doctor came in, introduced himself and asked Bernie if he knew who I was. Bernie smiled and whispered, 'Betty Lee.' Through it all, there was that smile, the smile I fell in love with, that smile that was just for me because he knew that 'Betty Lee' was there.

I talked with the doctor about his meds, his 'progress,' which I couldn't see, but he assured me that they could get Bernie stabilized. I sure didn't see how, but I had to let them try. What were my options?

I told Bernie that Debby had gone back to France, and he asked me about Matt's work, so he wasn't all that deeply medicated. He kept closing his eyes, trying to rest his head, and I just talked, tried to ease his head for him, and held his hand for a while.

He was silent for some time and then he whispered, "Don't give up on me." Crack! There went my heart again. I told him I wouldn't give up on him, promised I wouldn't give up on him. But it was an empty promise. I didn't know of anything else to do, anywhere else to turn, anyone else to ask. I felt as empty as I knew my promise to be.

Finally, I was escorted out through all the locked areas again, got into my car, drove to another gate that mysteriously opened by itself, retraced my treads on the freeway and went home to wait--that's what I did--wait.

72-HOUR HOLD	14-DAY HOLD	REFEREE
LEGALITIES	CONFINEMENT	KEYS
CONSERVATORSHIP	SECURITY	GUARD
ELOPEMENT	WALKIE-TALKIE	ADVOCATE

No, never, never did I think it would come to this.

"The Cuckoo's Nest"

"One Flew Over the Cuckoo's Nest"
Ken Kesey, 1962

It sounded so dramatic to say it, but I couldn't help it. This, then was madness. Insanity. We don't use those terms anymore, but that's what it was. The cuckoo's nest. Well, technically, medically speaking, I didn't really know. But that's what it seemed like to me. If medications weren't available to stabilize Bernie and violent people like him, that's exactly what we'd say. They're mad, they're insane, they're crazy. They'd have to be in padded cells, strapped down, in straitjackets, anything to keep them from hurting themselves and others. Oh, and much, much worse. I didn't even want to imagine what would happen to Bernie if the meds ever stopped being effective. So for now, his symptoms were controlled, but somewhere, someplace in the world, others must be out of control.

Calling it Alzheimer's instead of madness, crazy or insanity doesn't change what the patient goes through, but it does give us, hopefully, better understanding. Yet, even with understanding, we can't just let people go wild. Call their condition 'milk and honey' if you like, but patients still have to be controlled one way or another.

I well remember Bernie's telling me he wouldn't go into an insane asylum; he'd fight with every bit of his strength to keep from going into one--but God in heaven--I thought he was about as close to being in one as he could get. He was wholly out of control, his actions were insane. He'd be horrified if he knew some of the things he'd been doing.

We live in a time when we know what's wrong with people like this, I'd be more grateful if it were the future when, undoubtedly, there will be cures and prevention. I've thought of people like Bernie who lived generations ago when no one knew what was wrong, and didn't know what to do with them. Probably thought they were possessed, and that couldn't have been good either--exorcisms. And then there were lobotomies, shock treatments, snake pits, and more. All those horrors and terror. Poor souls.

Almost from the beginning of this nightmare, I'd had the feeling that Bernie had a certain prescience, as if he knew what was coming. He must have had the idea that he'd eventually be put into an insane asylum, otherwise, why mention it? How could he stand it, knowing that he was going mad? No wonder he talked about suicide.

Sometimes he seemed to read my mind, commenting about something I was only thinking and had never verbalized. Of course, he knew me quite well, so it may have been nothing more than familiarity, but at times, it seemed like more than that to me, like he just knew things.

And so there he was, my poor love, in a lockup. You'd never know, just by looking, what the place really was. Actually, it was pretty up there, located on a rise with a view of the city. Grounds were well maintained, lots of greenery, quiet, and outside tables where the staff could eat. The buildings were clean, it was nice, but still a place of forced confinement. A modern sanitized Bedlam.

My poor love.

It's Different Now

In the beginning I didn't ever ask for a prognosis, deliberately avoided the subject with doctors, and turned people off when they brought it up. What was the point? The last thing I wanted was to keep track on a mental calendar of how much time we had left together, to try to stuff everything we could think of into some sort of prescribed future time limit. Each day was enough, thank you.

But since I had placed him at Royale, everything changed. I knew that we were never going to be together again. Now, for several reasons, a prognosis became important to me, even though I knew it couldn't be absolutely accurate. After all, I couldn't even know how long I was going to live.

Like most diseases, there were parameters of Alzheimer's, but each patient was different. I'd heard of people dying in six months or just two years, while others lived indefinitely, 25 years or more. Bernie was doing well enough until three months earlier, and that was five years after diagnosis plus at least two or three years before that when I noticed subtle changes in him--which brings us to the seven-year, most common end to Alzheimer's, although I never felt he'd actually been diagnosed with that specific disease. But what else was there to call it now? So who knows?

In the past three months he'd been snowballing downhill faster than I could keep up--almost a daily decline. When I asked, the doctor said it's possible that Bernie could live for several years, maybe ten. Physically he was still in good health, but I wondered how much more his body could take. To me, it was under constant assault, plus all the meds.

What Now?

Bernie roamed the halls, walked into the rooms of other patients and got into their beds at night. He was scaring them, and he was still combative. The doctor was trying different drugs and placing him in 'Seclusion.' I just love these euphemisms.

Within days, the new meds were affecting his liver--and not really helping anyway--so now he was going to be on something else, but I didn't even bother to write it down. I had closed my drug book to all of it. I wasn't about to challenge these new meds, I had nothing better to offer. He was where he was, and I was where I was. I'd reached the plateau of the inevitable.

"Take Me Home"

The next time I saw Bernie he was tied into a wheelchair, wearing a diaper, and so bent over his nose was all but in his navel. When he realized I was beside him, he whispered, "Take me home." I told him I would, but, of course, I couldn't, although that's what I desperately wanted to do.

Of all the things for Bernie to clearly remember, why did it have to be 'home'? I could feel his ache to be home, to walk through the familiar rooms, to lie in his own bed beside me. I'd have given almost anything to bring him home, to let him rest there again, to sink into the comfort of the love, the contentment, and the safety he'd known there, but I didn't see how I could. Even worse, if I did, how could I ever take him back to a care facility again, once he'd been home? I just couldn't do it.

Oh, please, I begged with my heart, let him forget that part of his life already, let him remember something insignificant--a store, a restaurant, the barber shop--anything, but let him forget about home.

I was beginning to wonder if it was good for me to visit so often, but I just couldn't seem to stay away. My need for us to still touch was too powerful--well, what could you expect after half a century? And in recent days I'd grown even closer to him, had more of a need to be with him, to comfort him. I swear I'd sit and hold him all day if it was possible.

I remembered past times when I turned him away and fantasized that it would be different now, I'd be so much nicer, appreciate him more--but I knew nothing would change--not really. It's just that he was so vulnerable. I wanted to make up for every single slight, apologize for every anger, tell him how dear he's always been to me. But even if I talked to him about it now, told him how I wished we could do it all over again, how much better I'd be, I knew he couldn't understand. We were who we were, evenly matched, people said, and I wouldn't want to have changed that. Only now I couldn't get it into my head that I was really going to lose him. Although, in truth, I already had lost him.

•SIXTEEN•

It Worked!

Honestly, I never thought they could do it. I was going over the worst case scenario, knew Bernie wouldn't get better, just knew--but I was wrong.

They took him back to Royale by ambulance, all friendly, thanking the drivers, telling them he really enjoyed it, saying they should do it again soon. He ate all of his dinner, seemed to recognize some of the people, and was just as nice and friendly as could be. I was astonished--and pleased.

On the phone, I asked about Scottie. Hannah said she had a new boyfriend, in fact, she always had several. I was hoping she'd welcome Bernie back, help him settle in, to feel comfortable. Now it turned out she was just a fickle little hussy! Matt teasingly called her 'the trollop.'

When I went out to visit, I had no idea what to expect, but wasn't too surprised to see him in the lounge with Scottie, after all, sitting next to him on a couch, thigh to thigh. I guess she still preferred him. Dano separated them and brought Bernie to me in the hall.

I wasn't prepared for what happened next--oh, I was not at all prepared! He grabbed me and began smothering me with kisses. Big old-fashioned, hungry, smooching kisses. I didn't mind being kissed, but we were in a very public place with dozens of people milling around. Most of the patients near us wouldn't know or understand what was happening, and staff members understood, but I was really uncomfortable--really, really uncomfortable. He, on the other hand, was completely oblivious to our surroundings and anyone else. He was focused completely on me and what he was doing. I felt I had to get control.

Wiggling away, I led him to his room where he closed the drapes and began kissing me again--doing what guys do. He pulled me down on the bed and we laid there engaged in some serious necking. But at Royale, people walk in and out of the rooms all the time so I was even more uncomfortable.

I didn't want things to go any further. Could this be a side effect of the new medications? I had no idea what any side effects might be--if this could be called a 'side effect.' He certainly appeared stronger and healthier than when I'd last seen him, or maybe Scottie got him aroused. Hannah told me she often sits on his lap and kisses him.

It was almost lunchtime. If he didn't show up in the dining room I knew someone would soon come looking for him, so I suggested we go eat. He agreed and immediately forgot what he'd been doing.

I left him in the dining room eating with Scottie. On the way out, I stopped to tell Hannah what had happened. I was concerned that Bernie would turn into a 'dirty old man,' might approach one of the patients or a female visitor. But they had been through it all before. Don't worry she told me. If it happens, someone will sit with him and calm him down.

"Hard Would be Easy"

In the past, I've been as guilty as anyone else in offering platitudes to people--but sometimes, what else can one do? So I got a lot of them, not the least of which was, "What can I do to help?" Sadly enough, there really wasn't anything anyone could do, at least not at the moment.

Another favorite was, "It must be hard," or "I can imagine how hard it must be." Well, yeah, but probably not in the way people thought. The only thing that was really, really hard, was seeing Bernie go through all of this. The torture, the fear, the decline, the confusion, the mental and physical changes and deterioration--watching your loved one, seeing it on his face and body, in his eyes--it was so far beyond hard, that it made 'hard' look easy.

It was overwhelming, stupefying. It left me inert, disoriented, like I'd been through a giant bread slicer, sometimes unable to function. And that was just for openers. I knew more would be coming and there wasn't a thing I could do about it, other than to be there, to stand by, to comfort, to love, to take it, to take it, to take it, and to know that I'd stay with him, because that's what I wanted to do, and to get through it.

Things that others assumed were hard, really weren't for me. I didn't mind living alone, being alone, although I'd certainly prefer that Bernie was with me. We were supposed to grow old together, well, anyway, older than what we were, and I never thought that we should be completely immune to sorrow. In fact, we'd had a lot more happiness than many, I wasn't complaining--but---

I always seemed to be searching for elusive words to express the profound emptiness I felt at losing the one person who had loved me completely, unconditionally all my life. As annoyed and angry and disappointed as I had sometimes been with him, I always knew that Bernie would be there. I was a million miles from perfect, but it didn't matter to him. He just loved me.

I felt such conflict because he was still very much in my life, much more than I was in his. Of course, I always knew that he would probably, eventually forget me. But I never expected that I'd be replaced by others, strangers in a world where I didn't fit in. After a lifetime of being the center of his life, it was a little disconcerting to be left out in the cold, and to believe that he may not even think about me anymore.

The little bump-up from the meds only lasted a matter of days. Soon his head was lowered again and once more it was hard to get him to look at me, although he'd sometimes smile when he realized I was there. I wanted to knock on his crown and say, "Hey, pay attention, I'm still here." I was hungry for him to express his love like he used to, and sometimes he did, a bit here, a bit there, but it just wasn't the same, and it was hard to realize that that love didn't exist anywhere in the universe anymore. I missed it the way I would miss my warm coat if I'd left it in a restaurant, and then found that it wasn't there when I went back for it. I couldn't stop looking for it, it had to be someplace, and I was cold.

The Waiting Game

Matt went with me to see Bernie and he was much worse. He was sitting alone in the lounge, picking again at imaginary mites on the arm of his chair. We went right up to him, put our faces in front of his, but he wasn't able to focus on us, although I thought he knew who we were.

Bernie had been through such horror and terror, knowing and not knowing what was happening to him, that losing his awareness was more of a blessing than not. I almost had a sense of relief knowing it would happen.

Together then, each of us holding an arm in support, Matt and I walked him between us around the hallway. His steps were small, flat-footed, slow. When we asked him something, he barely muttered.

He was completely out of it. I asked Hannah if it was the meds doing it or the progress of the disease and she said it was not the medicine. He was also 'sundowning,' getting extremely agitated at the end of the day. She said that he'd lash out at others; he was extremely strong and difficult to control. They were thinking of increasing his medication.

September 3, 1998

"...Gone, Gone with the Wind ..."

"Cynara" 1896
Ernest Dowson

These are the words Margaret Mitchell chose for her epic work chronicling the postbellum South. She took them from her favorite poem, "Cynara," about a man's desolation and despair at losing his beloved to tuberculosis, because she said, "It had that far away, faintly sad sound I wanted."

That was pretty much my mood as I remembered that Bernie and I were married September 3, 1950, in the little two-bedroom corner house in Los Angeles where I grew up. My parents were second and third generation Americans, I was the last of three girls, living alone at home with them, still in grade school, while my sisters were already married and mothers; Bernie's parents were Hungarian born, and he was the sixth child of four boys and four girls. His family fascinated me. There were always people around, things going on--all those sisters and brothers. And by the same token, he really liked my family. He'd come over for dinner and my mother said she could never fill him up. Young boys eat a lot, but he never put on weight.

Everything Bernie did was a wonderment to me, maybe because I had no brothers. I used to fantasize that I was four inches high and stood in his shirt pocket all day, peeking out over the top like Kilroy, watching everything he did and going everywhere he went.

Do you hear all those 'clunk, clunks'? That's the sound of feminists fainting dead away at such thoughts. But I always thought that feminism just meant not having artificial barriers placed in our way, that we should have equal pay, education, and opportunity. I didn't think it meant we should try to change biology.

Every so often, some dipstick writes that we females shouldn't be so concerned about our appearance, our clothes, our hair. We shouldn't allow ourselves to become sex objects.

Oh, dear, dear, dear. The problem with such shallow reasoning, you see, is that in the real world, we are Sex Objects, that's why we're here. We naturally preen for men--and that's why they're here, to ogle us, to catch us. Now don't go having a hissy-fit--I didn't say that was the only thing we could or should do--I'm just saying that Nature has put us here to procreate (although we can control that now) and doesn't much care if we're lawyers, painters, or beachcombers while we're doing it. Don't challenge me; I didn't make up the rules.

All of this is by way of saying that I simply wanted to be with Bernie. I always loved him in spite of some really difficult times between us, and one of the reasons I loved him is because he let me be me--most of the time, and I let him be him.

Riding in his shirt pocket was a fantasy, not my reality, and I knew the difference. I've always been involved in things that had nothing to do with Bernie. But he was my rock, and I was his. Of course, not everyone wants that. People fly off in all directions all the time, but this is the way Bernie and I were. I was happy, and I believe he was, too. That's a lot to have--happiness.

I still loved Bernie, deeply and truly. But as time went on and we were no longer together, I was beginning to think that I loved the memories of our love, because there was no longer anything reciprocal. Still, I didn't think those memories could ever die, not for me, so I guess the 'Forever' engraved inside of our wedding rings, which neither of us ever wore, will forever mean 'forever.'

But I told Debby and Matt that from now on, September 3 would be just another day on the calendar. Please don't wish me 'Happy Anniversary.' A wedding anniversary isn't something that one can reasonably be happy to celebrate alone.

As I saw Bernie deteriorate physically and mentally, I still recognized the physical side of him that I so loved, but his essence that I equally loved was like a vapor that I could see but not touch, it no longer had a definitive form. I knew he desperately didn't want to go away, I knew he held onto me for dear life, but over the past few years, the past few months especially, he simply left me. And as his desperate fight mercifully appeared to be ending, almost willingly it seems, he moved into a personal mist where I could not follow, and there--he simply left me.

October 1998

Alzheimer's Association Walk

I had to do something substantial--something--so I contacted everyone I knew and asked them to donate to the Alzheimer's Association Walk in honor of Bernie. Of course, he'd know nothing about it, but I knew it was important. I was pleased and surprised when several family members showed up to walk with me.

Often little notes came with the donations--so touching, so poignant--and I'd sit at the kitchen table opening the envelopes, barely able to read through my tears. I had a goal of $1,000--but I raised $3,750!

"Married Widow"

I was supposed to go to the doctor every six to eight weeks to keep track of my blood pressure, but time got away from me and I hadn't been for five or six months. Finally, though, with Bernie more or less settled at Royale, I had the mental and emotional wherewithal to see the doctor. He was well aware of my being a sole caregiver and the stress that caused. Still, I was surprised when he asked me if I felt like a widow.

I didn't know what a widow was supposed to feel like. On the other hand, I certainly didn't feel married anymore--it was as if I had become a married widow, if there could be such a thing. People had been suggesting that I start dating other men. But, I didn't know about that, and I certainly didn't know where to find them anyway.

I felt like a wallflower everyone was passing by at the high school dance. I wanted to stop them and say, "Talk to me, smile at me, ask me to dance. I have a lot to offer." The problem, as I saw it, was that my world was now full of competing wallflowers and I was sure each one had a lot to offer. Maybe it was all just so new. The world didn't seem to be terribly enchanted with me. How come other men, unlike Bernie, just passed me by? I hadn't changed. But Bernie was still very much in my heart, my life, he was there, but really he wasn't there, and neither was anyone else. I thought my status made people uncomfortable.

So all in all, I really preferred to be by myself. Then I didn't have to pretend, to hold up, knowing that everyone would eventually leave anyway. They all had their own lives to live. I also had mine, but it was too shattered. I didn't feel free to pick up the pieces. I just felt much better off alone.

Visiting

My visits to Bernie were getting more and more difficult for me. Sitting with him in the lounge, holding his hand, he was mostly unaware of my presence. I asked him if he knew who I was and he muttered, I thought, about my being the prettiest girl in the room. I asked if he wanted to kiss me, and he pecked dutifully at my cheek. So somewhere he still had some understanding of who I was, but he was not really with me.

Scottie came over, touched his arm and he looked up and smiled. They began chattering together. To me, it sounded like a foreign tongue, I couldn't understand a thing they said, then she left. A moment later, Hannah came over, took his hands and he looked up and smiled broadly at her, too. He simply glowed, but he never did that with me anymore. She said that he talked about me all the time, but how she knew with his garbled speech, I couldn't say. He still introduced Scottie as his wife Betty, called her Betty, but all in all, the whole thing sucked.

I felt like a bystander, intrusive. I still wanted to see him, and I had to keep visiting anyway to see that he was being well cared for, but in truth, I had become an outsider.

My forty minute freeway drive, each way, could sometimes turn into an hour and I had been constantly expanding too much energy. I knew I had to back off. I could do much of his care on the phone. I'd call to see that he got his flu shot and his hair cut, or an appointment with the podiatrist, things like that. Otherwise, there wasn't much more for me to do. Royale always kept me informed about things he needed or problems he had. I'd go out once a week or so, I hoped that would be enough.

October 1998

Another Visit

Bernie doesn't know who I am.

◆ ◆ ◆

DEBBY

You give birth to this astonishing little person with such a quiet nature; your years are spent keeping her safe, and in less than an ethereal nanosecond she becomes an understanding adult, accepting of so many difficult things you need to tell her, a confidant never too busy to listen, an emotional support you can always count on--a daughter.

JEAN-FRANÇOIS

If ever a son-in-law went above and beyond the call of duty, it is this man. I will always be grateful for everything he did during that special interlude we spent together. It was so stressful, so heart-wrenching, and--so damn funny.

ZELI

Without qualification, Zeli simply loved Bernie. She was the one who watched him when I had to go out, picked him up from day care when I couldn't, too often cleaned up his accidents; and most importantly, never put her husband between herself and his parents when they needed him--a rare woman, indeed.

ESTELLA

Zeli's mom, Estella, is everything that a mother-in-law can be--and more. She, too, watched Bernie when Zeli was at work and there were things I had to do. She also helped clean him up, always made something yummy and tasty for him to eat, did his mending and sewed countless name tags on his clothes--a joyful gift.

HARRY

"Our lives are like the course of the sun. At the darkest moment there is the promise of daylight."

London 'Times' Editorial
December 24, 1984

AUTHOR'S NOTES

When Bernie and I began this sad sojourn, I had no idea that it would create such outrageous, destructive changes in our lives, much less that I'd find myself embroiled in the middle of a medical controversy that would jolt me awake to people and things I really didn't want to know about. If I've learned anything, it's the fundamental truths that 'no good deed goes unpunished,' and 'there are none so blind as those who will not see.'

There are two concurrent stories now--(1) Bernie's progression; and (2) the consequence of what I did to help him. Because some insist on calling what happened controversial--it isn't--I have changed almost all names and locations or left them out completely, literally to shield those who don't need any more aggravation about it. Exceptions are Dr. Goldsmith, Brian and Helen Sternberg, Drew Griffin, Larry Greene, and UCLA.

My medical knowledge is that of an ordinary layman. Some came from school, being a mom, taking care of myself or others, some specific outside reading from time to time, labels and inserts, a home medical book and drug guide, questions to doctors, living life, but it's all pretty superficial.

I do have a fundamental understanding of what I've written here, (learned the hard way), but believing that most people are like me and don't know all that much about the medical technicalities of Alzheimer's, I've tried to make it easy to follow. There are some technical words that you might have to look up--maybe some questions for a doctor--but the gist is there, as clear as I could make it.

Nonetheless, there are those who will dismiss what happened, call me a silly gullible old woman, the doctor a fraud, and on and on with no proof whatsoever of their baseless nattering. But everything is documented. Much of it remains on the Internet, on videos both televised and private, in hospital records, medical publications and on papers in my office. I never had to make up anything--it was all just bizarre enough as it happened.

(*) Indicates 'Finding References' on Page 356.

"See there's this place in me where your fingerprints still rest, your kisses still linger, and your whispers softly echo. It's the place where a part of you will forever be a part of me."

Gretchen Kemp

◆SEVENTEEN◆

December 1998

Seattle, Washington

Only weeks ago, our lives had finally settled and stabilized. Bernie, having been returned to Royale Park no longer knew me, and I felt it would be OK to leave him for a bit, maybe a trip to France; but instead, Matt and I were staring at the waters lapping around the dock of a Seattle yacht club. Soon we'd be inside, having lunch with strangers, hoping against hope once again that something would come of this, that a minor miracle may be in the offing, even though I'd promised myself I wouldn't be chasing any more rainbows.

It began with an article about new drugs and hope for Alzheimer's by a medical reporter in a Sunday supplement magazine in the Los Angeles Times. I wasn't going to read it. I knew about the new drugs and had very little faith in any long-term effects. All the hype, all the exciting 'breakthroughs' went nowhere for me. This article was just another media filler in an endless stream of Alzheimer's stories, my search was over, the end, *adios*, finished, *fini, kaput, aloha, arrivederci, sayonara,* get outta my face, don't bother me anymore. In no small measure, I was content with my decisions and what I had done. It wasn't what I'd planned, certainly not what I'd wanted, but nonetheless, here it was and I was OK with it. You know, if life hands you lemons, make lemonade. Well, I'd made so much lemonade I should have been drowning in it. Instead, I was still floating--struggling, to be sure, but still afloat, just as I'd promised my family and myself.

But I read the article anyway and there, incredibly, I found something new, something I didn't understand at all, some sort of mysterious surgery.

It reported that in the summer of 1998 at an International Conference on Alzheimer's Disease in Amsterdam, there had been a presentation by a Dr. Harry S. Goldsmith of the University of Nevada School of Medicine, who had performed this surgery on a 65-year-old minister's wife from Texas with severe brain atrophy who could no longer speak or feed herself. This Dr. Goldsmith had developed a procedure that uses the patient's own omentum, a biochemical-rich membrane in the abdomen, and places it on the brain! Six months after she had surgery in Germany, the woman was more alert, spoke a little, sang along with hymns, recognized people and laughed appropriately when listening to conversations.

"These are little things, but at this stage you take what you can get, and you cherish it," said her daughter. By golly, I agreed, and I'd be thrilled to take that over what I *knew* was coming! Further, an autopsy on a previous patient, who had died from unrelated causes two and a-half years after the same surgery, showed that signs of Alzheimer's in the brain had been reduced. I had no idea what this was all about, but I was darn sure going to find out. I turned on my computer.

What's an Omentum, anyway?

My 1977 Edition of *Gray's Anatomy* described the 'lesser omentum,' the 'greater omentum,' and the 'gastro-splenic omentum.' They are located near the stomach, seem to contain a variety of blood vessels, and *"the use of the great omentum appears to be to protect the intestines from the cold, and to facilitate their movement upon each other during their vermicular* (pertaining to, or done by worms) *action."* Well, OK, but that's the wrong part of the body, what does it have to do with the brain?

My computer search offered little about the omentum itself. Most medical dictionaries or medical Web sites didn't even mention it, and when it did appear, it was vaguely described as a biochemical-rich membrane in the abdomen, just as reported in the article, but nothing about what those biochemicals were or what further purpose the omentum had, much less how it might help Alzheimer's. There was a little more in an encyclopedia that said it was a double membrane that hangs from the stomach and is one of the major fat-storage areas in the body, which may finally explain that little pouch so many of us try to suck in.

I did find a surgical procedure called *omentum (or omental) transposition.* But instead of finding out about Alzheimer's, I just kept reading about spinal cord injuries, of all things. From time to time I'd find something about stroke victims having the surgery, so there was some connection to the brain--but I still didn't get it.

It would be a while before I learned what the connection was. Essentially, our brain and spinal cord make up our central nervous system. All the other nerves in our body make up the peripheral nervous system. Obviously the two systems communicate with each other, but when there is a breakdown in the central nervous system, either from an accident or medical condition, the messages can't get out to the peripheral nerves. This causes all sorts of physical and brain malfunctions, and if severe enough, lack of function altogether. The problem then becomes how to repair the trauma to the central nervous system. There are many possible solutions; medications, therapies, or surgeries. This particular surgery, applying the omentum to the trauma, would hopefully restore blood flow. Not everything works for every patient every time, but Bernie's condition was too destructive to dismiss any possibility out of hand without thorough investigation, so I thought omentum transposition was an idea with merit that deserved closer inspection--and I still thought about blood flow.

I posted on an omentum message board, asking for anyone to tell me 'good or bad' if they knew about the surgery. The only response I got was one telling me it was dangerous and to stay away from it. When I asked what the dangers were, I never heard back. I wasn't happy about that--someone got me all frightened and riled up, playing with my head--gave me an empty warning and then went mute. Not a good sign.

At one Web site about spinal cord injuries, I found a brief excerpt from the magazine article about the Alzheimer's patient mentioned in Amsterdam, but nothing further. I'd find negative reports about Dr. Goldsmith at other sites and, of course, followed them up. They all turned out to be garbage spin. What was going on? Finally I decided to go to the source and tracked down the reporter who had written the piece.

The Source

I found her in New York and talked her ears off. She told me that she had followed Dr. Goldsmith around the world for 18 months, thought he was terrific, and was at the Amsterdam conference when he had presented the paper about the Texas woman. When the conference was ending, a group of reporters and doctors sat around discussing what was newsworthy enough to release to the media. She suggested Dr. Goldsmith and omentum surgery, but was told, essentially, that while they all thought Dr. Goldsmith was a nice enough man, no one took him and his work all that seriously and they preferred to publicize other things.

Later she did try to write about Dr. Goldsmith, gave potential material to her agent, but wherever they tried, anything about him or his work in any form was always turned down. She knew the gossip I'd found about him on the Internet and the opposition to his work, so when she wrote the article I'd read, she decided to try to sneak in a few lines about the surgery, hoping the editors wouldn't notice, but that someone reading it would follow up. Meanwhile, she had located and kept in contact with the family of the Texas woman who was the subject of Dr. Goldsmith's presentation, and while the woman would never be her old self, she was better and continued to do well.

I understood that the reporter had no ax to grind, no possible financial gain; she was just trying to get the word out about something she believed could help people. It appeared all straightforward to me, and why she had to use subterfuge to publish such important information seemed bizarre. Thinking about her background and knowledge of the medical field--which I certainly didn't have--I took what she said to heart and, in spite of the negative comments on the Internet, decided to continue my research on the omentum and contact Dr. Goldsmith.

Learning Through Surprise

Of all places, I found out a lot about the omentum at South Paws, (http://www.southpaws.com), a veterinary referral center. It explained that the omentum is a unique and versatile organ that can be utilized for a variety of procedures. Along with having glucose and all our other necessary biological agents, (or in this case, a dog's), it is a source of blood vessels! There it was, right there, being used on puppies and kittens, a way to increase diminished blood flow! Why wouldn't it work on Bernie? It had to, it just had to. It had already worked on the brains of other people.

The article went on to describe how the omentum could be lengthened and utilized in surgeries involving nearly all parts of the animal's body. It could also assist in chronic, non-healing skin wounds by tunneling it under the skin to the wound site and suturing it into place, and it was used in the absorption of fluids in a number of body locations, something I did understand and knew to be important. The article ended: *"The omentum is an extremely useful organ with a variety of potential uses. Clearly, it was placed in the abdomen for a reason. The best rule of thumb, then, is to go ahead and utilize it when you can."* That was good news, indeed, but do cats and dogs get Alzheimer's? A ten-year-old dog would be 70, so maybe. I knew that distemper affects a dog's brain, but I didn't think it was the same thing. Anyway, now that I had a glimmer of how it worked, I was really beginning to believe that it would help, so I kept on searching.

Over the years, I'd heard of Buerger's Disease (http://www.worldmedics.com/vkagarwal), but I never knew anyone who had it, although I knew that people with Buerger's could lose their legs because the blood flow is cut off. But omentum transposition surgery brings revascularization to the leg--all the way to the toes--

and in four to eight days circulation develops and the leg is saved. Again, I didn't understand all the details, but I sure understood that. As with dogs, it is fortuitous that the omentum is so centrally located in the body--if it could reach our toes, obviously it could reach our brains--but how?

At (http://www.ncbi.nlm.nih.gov/entrez), (this address goes to the U.S. Government Web site for the National Center for Biotechnology Information, National Library of Medicine, and the National Institutes of Health), the reader can type 'omentum transposition' into 'search,' where there are all sorts of examples of omentum transposition uses, including how it is used after cardiac and mastectomy surgeries, on liver cysts, cerebral infarctions, Alzheimer's, and pages of other applications I didn't understand.

Checking Further

While all of that was very interesting, there was still very little about Alzheimer's, so I called the Chicago Headquarters of the Alzheimer's Association and asked what they thought about omentum transposition. The full and complete answer they gave me was, "You'll have to find the doctor on your own." Of course, I already knew who the doctor was, but what I understood from their response was that they also knew who the doctor was, what the surgery was, and that they weren't about to help me. That left me up in the air. If they knew about it and if they thought it was useless and the doctor was a quack, wouldn't they tell me? I'd already gone to (http://www.quackwatch.com), and there was nothing there on Dr. Goldsmith, so what was going on here?

The magazine article had also mentioned the Ronald & Nancy Reagan Research Institute, maybe they'd know something about it and so I called and spoke to the Director. Yes, he knew about it, but didn't know enough to say 'yea or nay.' I appreciated the man's honesty; at least no one dismissed me, and he didn't have anything negative to say about Dr. Goldsmith either. I didn't know all the medical ethics about such things, maybe they just don't talk about each other. Anyway, it was all good. I'd spoken directly to an insider who didn't reject the surgery, so I felt confident now to make my own decision about it. I said I was thinking about having it done for my husband and asked if he'd like me to report back afterwards. He said he'd be interested, and I took that to be a positive note.

But just to make sure, I checked him out, too. He had published several books on Alzheimer's and at one time appeared to focus in on dementia postmortem, so he was in the thick of it, was with an organization of some prestige and I trusted what he told me. After all, this was Bernie's life.

An Astonishing Discovery

Then I discovered the most fascinating thing--the actual report of the first patient's autopsy that was mentioned in the reporter's story, titled "Decreased Senile Plaque Density in Alzheimer Neocortex Adjacent to an Omental Transposition" (*) written by Dr. Goldsmith and four other doctors. It had been published August 1996, in *Neurological Research*. Why hadn't I heard about all of this? I'd certainly been to enough doctors, surely they knew about it. They read journals, talk to each other, or at least they should. Wouldn't you think the news would spread like wildfire? Instead, it was apparently being squelched for people while veterinarians were using it successfully on animals--for goodness sakes!

The autopsy report had photographs of brain tissue that showed plaques in the brain had been reduced where the omentum was placed compared to the section without it. Of course I didn't know what I was looking at, but clearly there appeared to be a substantial change of something going on from one photograph to the other. One looked like an overabundant starry night sky, while the other looked like a very skimpy starry night sky--an obvious difference between the two.

Surgery was done at an east coast university by Dr. Goldsmith in March 1993, and yet, here it was, over five years later and no one seemed to be doing anything about it! Obviously it could alleviate a lot of misery, so why not?

A companion article "Comment on Omental Transposition for Alzheimer's Disease," (*) related that neurologists at an Ivy League University had followed the patient's improved neurological and mental status from surgery until his death.

It further referred to the theory of Alois Alzheimer (1854-1915), the German doctor the disease is named for, and who published a monumental work on the subject in 1907. It read:

"...having been mentioned in passing by Alois Alzheimer himself shortly after his description of the disorder that bears his name, Alzheimer thought that reduced cerebral perfusion could be the cause of the pathologic lesions that formed in the brain of his patients but did not give a reason for this conclusion."

The article continued, *"An extension of Alzheimer's concept is the hypothesis which maintains that the metabolic dysfunction and cellular holocaust developing in Alzheimer brains over many years is due to the slow starvation of sensitive neurons unable to keep pace with the normal metabolic energy demand resulting from a reduced micronutrient energy delivery. This neuronal starvation would be partly complicated by the reduced cerebral blood flow seen in these patients but more specifically, it would result from a structurally impaired cerebral capillary system that is unable to meet the energy demand required by the affected neurons."* In layman's words, I took that to mean diminished blood flow may well be a culprit in Alzheimer's. It further cited animal studies that bolster the theory, and noted that substantial clinical evidence has for many years indicated that chronic cerebral hypoperfusion is one of the most significant factors associated with brain dysfunction.

So I thought back to 1993, that Dr. Franklin knew what he was talking about when he told me Bernie's short-term memory loss was because of diminished blood flow in his brain, and if I could get this surgery done and increase the blood flow, there was a darn good chance it would help, although I wasn't sure just how, but I couldn't see that it would hurt either. I knew it was only a matter of time until I'd lose him; any substantial improvement seemed worth the gamble.

My medical background is strictly that of a lay-person, and I know that a little knowledge can be a dangerous thing, but common sense and simple logic always underlie everything that works. If it's a sound theory, you can't change the basic premise, and what I was finding told me that it would work. Technical details can be left to the experts, but essentially, this is what I understood.

Somehow, during surgery, one end of the omentum is placed on the brain, new blood vessels form to bring blood into the brain, and blood brings oxygen. I understood the basic concept, that the omentum could bring blood to nourish the brain, I just didn't know how it was all done, and even knowing that it could reach the feet, it still seemed like a long stretch to get through the skull.

Something caused Bernie's blood vessels to constrict and that subsequent slowing of blood and oxygen nourishing the brain could have caused other damage. Whenever the blood supply to any part of the body is cut off, that part will eventually die, and that includes the brain. If it wasn't early aging, maybe it was some other unseen out of whack body chemistry that could have caused the constriction, maybe silent mini-strokes, stress, even a long-dormant recessive gene. Cells were dying, electrical impulses were going haywire. Which came first, the chicken or the egg? From our family doctor, through UCLA and on to several respected neurologists, none of them knew, so I'd certainly never know and by now, I couldn't have cared less anyway.

Dead cells could not be restored, no one was claiming that. But if we could by-pass the constriction, get fresh nourishment--blood and oxygen into the brain--it might slow down the dying off of some of the other cells. Blood flow was something I'd been looking for for years. The chelation and the oxygen chambers never helped, but here was another avenue that seemed more direct and far less 'iffy.'

It was something from his own body that might help him *now*, without drug side effects, no rejection and a good chance that any positive effects would last longer than the projected six or seven months I was told he might get from medications. Obviously surgery was a lot more radical than pills, but the brain is operated on routinely. If you were told that you had brain cancer and only six months to live unless you had brain surgery, most people would do it immediately. In a way, Bernie was in that same position, except that his prognosis was worse than dying, he could become a vegetable.

Finding Dr. Goldsmith

If you've been on a computer long enough, you discover the world is filled with a lot of wackos who are compelled to post whatever comes into their sick heads, sometimes it's quite vile. Once it's on the Internet, it's pretty much there forever, and if it's a packet of lies and distortions, there's little the victim can do about it. I still didn't know exactly who, how or why there seemed to be an obvious vendetta against this Dr. Goldsmith, but it was a horrible injustice for those patients who might have benefited from his skills, and it certainly was not a unique story in the medical field. People were being frightened away. Why would anyone do such a cruel thing?

If I were to believe all the nonsense about him on the Web, Dr. Goldsmith was some sort of snake oil scam artist hiding out in a cave someplace. One post said to report him to the authorities, but when I contacted the state police mentioned, they told me they'd never heard of him. It's not surprising that authorities haven't heard of someone who has, perhaps, never been reported. There was no further way that I could follow all of this, so I typed his name into my search engine and it immediately popped up with his phone number in Nevada. Either he was the dumbest fugitive in the country, or the authorities couldn't find their own backsides.

Still, I had to follow up everything negative that I'd read. There was supposed to be a "60 Minutes" segment about all the terrible things he and his 'agent' had done to spinal cord injury patients, but when I accessed the archives of "60 Minutes," I couldn't find any program about him--and I went back several years. I read that what was called a 'New England university' where he'd practiced surgery had closed down his clinic, but when I looked up the cited school, it turned out to be a culinary college in Florida. So maybe something had happened sometime, somewhere but I couldn't find it. I felt it was time to forget the whole sordid mess of gossip--whatever it was, I'd probably find out soon enough.

Making Contact

Dr. Goldsmith answered his phone personally. He listened to my story about Bernie and wanted to know if he'd had any abdominal surgery, especially cancer. He explained that if someone had cancer in the vicinity of the omentum, the omentum would be routinely removed because it is so rich that it feeds the cancer cells, and the patient had to have an omentum in order to have the surgery. Even if it wasn't cancer, if the surgery was too extensive, it could damage the omentum to the point where it wouldn't be usable. Bernie did have that colon surgery a few years back, but the polyp was benign and the scar wasn't all that big. Dr. Goldsmith said if I decided to do it, he'd come to Los Angeles and examine Bernie, but from what I described, he didn't think it would be a problem. Nonetheless, it gave me something to worry about because I was seriously thinking that I wanted Bernie to have this surgery--and I wanted the omentum intact.

There was a little more chitchat and he told me that he was giving a small presentation in a few days in Seattle about spinal cord injuries for one of his patients, Brian Sternberg. If I wanted to meet him, I'd be more than welcome, and that's how Matt and I found ourselves gazing out over Puget Sound.

Getting Acquainted

Brian Sternberg

I had a dim memory of Brian Sternberg as a world class athlete, and this luncheon was being hosted by his Kiwanis Club. They wanted to hear about Dr. Goldsmith's research and surgery for spinal cord injuries.

Reading some of his mother Helen's handouts about Brian told me more. Thirty-five years ago in 1963, at age 19, he was the world's number one pole vaulter and part of a United States team going to an upcoming competition in Russia. But in a trampoline accident just days before the event, he was left a quadriplegic, only able to move his shoulders. Helen spoke at length to Matt and me with nothing but praise for Dr. Goldsmith who had operated on her son two years ago--*33 years* after the injury!

Before the surgery, she told us, there was so much weakness in Brian's diaphragm that his voice, barely a whisper, couldn't be heard across a dining room table. He was pale, drawn, desperately thin and in such constant severe pain that nothing seemed to help. Once his reactions became so intense that they thought they were going to lose him. For over thirty years he lived in such pain that on a scale of 1 to 10, he said his pain was 8 to 13. Now, after surgery, it's down to 3. His voice is strong, he has more feeling in his fingers and toes, his circulation has greatly improved, and he can move his thumbs. His overall stamina has dramatically increased. Before he couldn't sit upright long enough to eat a meal, but on a recent auto trip from Seattle to Palm Springs he was able to sit quite a bit. In my view, the ability of the body to regain even a modicum of activity after so many years was incredible.

I never had a chance that afternoon to speak to Brian personally, but what I saw as he chatted with others was an imposing middle-aged man, charming, quite handsome, even distinguished looking. With assistance, he has always continued to work out physically and it shows, his body is that of a well-toned athlete. Helen said that little improvements still continue to happen, so they're looking forward to more--and why not?

A second patient, a woman, also along with her mother, had lunch with us at our table. Vibrant, dramatically beautiful, now 37 years old, she'd been struck by a drunk driver seven years earlier. Left a quadriplegic, she was unable to do anything other than lie in bed moving only her head from side to side. Now, after Dr. Goldsmith performed omentum surgery on her, she can use her right arm to feed and groom herself. She operates her own wheelchair, drives a specially equipped van, and has a job taking catalog orders. Yes, she can write. She delighted in telling us, with an apology, that the best thing is her being able to use the bathroom by herself. Her mother spends an hour each morning and each evening helping her; otherwise she's on her own.

The Slide Show

Good grief! Dr. Goldsmith's slide show presentation was a lot to take in. Although I could grasp the idea, and had personally witnessed the results, I'm not technically or medically equipped to go into accurate detail.

But the way I understood it, any number of conditions can interrupt blood flow and that leads to major problems. How to restore that circulation has always been a medical puzzle, but somewhere along the way Dr. Goldsmith set forth the idea that the omentum had the capacity to do just that. Decades ago he began animal experiments for spinal cord injuries and the slides were geared only to that, nothing about Alzheimer's. They showed the animal experiments, cats that had been unable to walk, details about the surgery, and then how they walked again. Eventually it was done on humans.

Simply put, an incision is made in the abdomen above the omentum releasing one end so that it can be surgically elongated. Leaving the blood vessels intact, and avoiding any vital organs, it is then fed under the skin to the site of the spinal cord injury where it is placed. In what appeared to me to be a sort of morphing, the omentum and the damaged spinal tissue melded or fused as the omentum began to offer itself to the injury. Tiny omentum blood vessels with all their precious biochemistry then dug into the damaged tissue in the same way tree roots burrow into the earth. How? Well, how would *I* know how?

Yes, it was a little icky when we saw the omentum being worked on, but then surgery is icky. While there was no improvement in about fifty percent of the patients, there was a wide range of improvement in the others, two of them sitting in the same room with me. It was enough to give me confidence in Dr. Goldsmith and the procedure--the odds were very good.

A Conundrum

Helen also told us the story and subsequent fallout about "60 Minutes," except that it wasn't "60 Minutes," it was another news magazine program. Since I wasn't involved at the time, I cannot verify the accuracy of anything she said, it's all hearsay and I won't be held accountable. So, right or wrong here it is, take it on faith or not.

For a couple of years, Boston University's medical center had been doing omental transposition surgeries on spinal cord injury patients who had all signed informed consents with the understanding that there was no guarantee they'd get better. Several patients, however, had been showing some improvements. Meanwhile, a woman who ran a physical therapy clinic in another state had taken some of her patients to the clinic to be operated on. One of her patients said that the woman was telling them that favorable results could be expected, although neither Dr. Goldsmith nor any of the other doctors involved made any such claims and did not know that anyone was making them.

The complaining patient never made any legal claim personally, but attorneys subsequently went to other patients who'd had the surgery and eventually got some of them to make complaints against several of the doctors and the hospital. Insurance companies, as is their too-often wont, chose to settle the claims rather than go to court, even though no wrongdoing was ever evidenced. Helen believed that the patients shown on television were not all that unhappy with their surgeries, but were made to look as if they were. She was so incensed that she even got her local television station to interview other omental surgery patients to refute what had been shown on television. On advice of legal counsel, Dr. Goldsmith declined to be interviewed for the show. It was thought he might be edited to make him look bad, and indeed, excerpts from previous talks he'd given appeared to do just that.

Everyone began suing everyone else and the university, although aware that neither any of the doctors nor the hospital had done anything wrong, felt that they had to shut down the project because they couldn't handle all the likely resulting legalities and expenses. They even refunded some patient fees rather than contest lawsuits. None of the suits against Dr. Goldsmith ever came to fruition. He sued the television station for defamation. A California law firm took his case on *pro bono,* but when the network had the case moved to Massachusetts where there would be no punitive damages rendered, and it would be dragged out for years and always running cross-country, the case was dropped.

So there was some veiled truth to the things I found on the Web after all, but why it was obviously disinformation, I cannot say. Nonetheless, stopping the surgeries prevented many spinal cord injury victims from getting the best chance they had at the time for any hope of improvement and Dr. Goldsmith's professional reputation was badly tarnished. He felt that his only option was to continue his work out of the public eye and let the brouhaha fade away.

There was a final report that stated he should have known an alleged misrepresentation about the surgery was being made by an unauthorized agent--a very strange concept--how can you know what you have no way of knowing? It sounded like a big legal, political, ratings-hungry, financially greedy mess of people and had nothing to do with the doctor's medical skills or ethical standards. In my view, it was just so much chaff to blow away.

I tried repeatedly to get a video or transcript of the program, but I never could. I was told it couldn't be done without a release from everyone who appeared on the tape and I didn't think that would be possible.

Until now Helen Sternberg didn't even know that Bernie existed, that I might want the surgery, she had nothing to gain if I did it or not, and so I trusted her, too, and I was more certain than ever that someone was out to get the doctor, to stop omentum transposition--but that was not my primary concern--my goal was to increase blood flow in Bernie's brain.

Matt and I couldn't help but be impressed by these people eager to share their experiences with us. More and more I felt that this is where I was meant to be--here in this strange place in a roomful of strangers who understood my quest and who held the key for my only hope to give Bernie a slim chance.

Stroke Victims

Ben and Cindy DeCarlo were also at our table. Ben had had a major stroke four years ago and was already scheduled to have omentum surgery in Germany. Only 61, he looked so healthy and moved so normally, I hardly believed that he'd suffered the massive stroke Cindy described, although having lost his language skills, his speech was belabored, and he'd lost his reading and writing abilities as well. Cindy had, also, done a lot of research on the omentum, and Ben's hope was that the surgery would restore some of his lost abilities.

They knew that his chance of improvement was again about fifty-fifty, but they felt with an increased blood supply to the brain, if nothing else, it would act as a barrier against another attack.

Ben had made the decision on his own to go to Germany. Although the procedure did not impact any major organs, and did not invade the brain, he knew full well it was still, in effect, a double surgery. But there's nothing unique about a double surgery, and now he saw a possibility to better his life, a chance, and he wasn't about to sit back and do nothing more effective than feel sorry for himself. They were flying to Germany in January--only a month away.

"He Who Saves One Life, Saves The World Entire"

The Talmud, as spoken in
"Schlinder's List" - 1993

Right after the slide show, everyone crowded around wanting to talk to Dr. Goldsmith. I'd elbow my way in, get elbowed away, and go back in again. When Matt and I were finally able to introduce ourselves, he seemed surprised that we'd actually flown up just for the day, but there we were, and we were interested.

He was about my age and pretty much looked and sounded like a Hollywood casting call for a low-key family physician who had spent too many hours at too many bedsides when he should have been asleep himself. But mention the omentum, and his eyes lit up like a neon sign. He was absolutely glommed onto it and all the miraculous things he believed it could do. I thought if he was discussing the omentum, and someone interrupted to tell him that he'd just won the lottery, he'd never miss a beat.

I've met other people like him. They can be so intense about one thing in life that almost everything else is crowded out. But that's the way it has to be if we are ever going to have progressive changes--some people just think outside the box--thank goodness--and while the rest of their community is telling them 'it's not possible,' they're already halfway there to figuring it out.

But Matt and I had to leave. I could phone and talk to him about Bernie when I got home. It was too noisy and crowded now, not a good time to discuss anything so important. Besides, we had a plane to catch and a lot to think about.

Why Not Try It?

If Bernie had the surgery, he'd be only the third Alzheimer's patient to do it, so there was really no way of assessing the percentage of success. Other than the risks that come with any medical procedure, I didn't think it was that risky compared to watching Bernie turn into a vegetable--and *those* percentages I did know.

Omentum transpositions are done in the United States but only for the occasional stroke victim and only at one or two select locations. Currently it is not done here for any other condition, including spinal cord injuries, and certainly not for Alzheimer's. There is no insurance coverage and it is substantially more expensive than the cost of having it done abroad, which is why patients go to Germany--that and because it's accepted there. It is done in several other countries for various conditions, especially in Southern China where it is performed mainly for strokes, encephalitis and cerebral palsy.

Since omentum transposition is a well-established procedure that has been around for decades, and repeatedly proven in practice, I can't understand why the American medical community chooses to turn a deaf ear and a blind eye to this option in the fight against Alzheimer's. I get asked that question all the time and my only answer is, "You'll have to ask them."

As with chelation, there are always those who will not abide anything new. If it hasn't been scientifically proven, anything positive is dismissed as anecdotal--as if anecdotal is bad. This 'must be scientifically proven' mantra is likely stifling many worthwhile procedures. Some people would be against aspirin if it came on the scene today. If it has never been proven scientifically effective, you can make the same argument that it has not been proven scientifically *ineffective* either. If double-blind studies are never done, then it can never be proven scientifically one way or the other, which leaves people like us hanging out to dry. But some things will never lend themselves to double-blind studies--and that's a fact. Although fake surgeries are done for some double-blind studies, in my opinion, doing it with omentum transposition for Alzheimer's is no more reasonable than doing it for heart transplants. That being the case, why not try it?

The vast majority of medical procedures currently practiced have never been scientifically proven. They've just come down through the generations, many improving over time as techniques and technology get better, but they had to start someplace. And, we, the public have an inherent right to study issues and make an informed, responsible decision about our own medical care--right or wrong--we have that right!

The Decision

In the end, the decision to have the surgery made itself. There's nothing unique about having brain surgery to save someone's life and Bernie's life was certainly worth saving. I knew from the very beginning I was going to do it and was completely comfortable about it. Even if Bernie died, which I didn't think for a minute would happen, he'd have lost nothing. He had talked about suicide more than once, he wasn't that much in love with life anymore, and I'd already lost him long ago.

When I first placed him at Royale Park, they told me that he'd probably last about three years, average for such care facilities. Then the doctor at the mental institution said it could be ten years, so no one really knew. And I had come to believe that the heavy sedation everyone kept prescribing was going to kill him sooner anyway. If drugs slowed down brain activity, they had to slow down the rest of his organs as well, though sometimes I thought it sped things up, but either way, it couldn't be good. It would be worth it just to get him off the meds.

But whatever time Bernie had left was not the issue, it was that he deserved better. If he was a lot older, he was only 69, or if there was an additional debilitating disease, I'd never consider it, but he was otherwise healthy and far too young to be left to exist like he was for untold years--not if there was even a remote chance of helping him. I simply couldn't not do it, to let him deteriorate, sliding rapidly downhill. The best thing was to get him to Europe while Dr. Goldsmith was already there operating on Ben DeCarlo the following month. I felt that every day I let go by hastened his decline. I wanted to do it *yesterday!*

Besides, I discovered I'd been badly mistaken about Bernie's not knowing me. When it happened, when he pushed me away, he was deeply sedated. In subsequent visits, made later in the day, when meds were wearing off, he'd been more alert, known Matt, Zeli, and me. That was a serious presumption on my part--and wrong.

◆EIGHTEEN◆

"No Gamble, No Gain"

As he promised, Dr. Goldsmith came to Royale Park to examine Bernie. He also wanted to make sure that Bernie understood what we were going to try to do. If he was wholly resistant, he couldn't be hog-tied and forced into an operating room.

I'd told Royale not to give Bernie his meds that day and asked Dr. Goldsmith to come in the late afternoon when he was most aware--if he was aware at all. I'd been told that if the drugs were stopped, their effects would still last for about three days, but he wouldn't be in such a deep stupor, and I knew it could take a long time for drugs to completely leave the system of some patients. But this was the best I could do.

Bernie's response to the doctor was his usual garbled gibberish, but with patience and much repeating, Dr. Goldsmith finally began to get through. He told him there was an operation that might help him regain some of his memory, but he didn't go into a lot of detail, it's hard enough for lucid people to comprehend this particular surgery.

At first Bernie backed away, defensive, and jabbered that he didn't want anyone cutting into his organs. But after a bit, as he realized he was talking to a doctor, he wanted to know why he was the way that he was, and I could see the old Bernie coming to the fore. I always believed that Bernie was still in there, that he knew what was happening, so I wasn't surprised when he wanted an explanation of 'why?' Then, as he had always done, he could analyze it and fix it.

Finally I saw him beginning to understand, to become involved in the conversation. For almost an hour the doctor had been slowly repeating that there was a chance for him to get better, telling him, honestly, that there were no guarantees. Then he said, "It's a gamble." Bernie immediately picked up on the word 'gamble.' He answered, "no gamble, no gain," and I knew we'd broken through, that he understood--he understood it was a gamble and he was willing to take it.

Arrangements For Germany

I'd been making arrangements for our trip to Germany and it was all but an endless task. Because you can't take a violent person on an airplane, Bernie would have to continue to be sedated and he'd need wheelchairs. I couldn't watch him and also take care of passports, luggage, tickets, boarding passes, and everything else, especially in large bustling, busy foreign airports, and you can only expect so much help from airline personnel.

Matt would go with me and stay until after the surgery. For our return flight, Jean-François would come from France, fly home with us and then go back to the Pyrenees the next day. I'd bought us all economy tickets, and because it was January, the costs were reasonable. I used all our frequent flyer mileage to upgrade us to Business Class and pretty much depleted our accounts. I didn't have enough miles left to fly to Catalina. But it had to be that way. In Business Class, we'd have more room, we could put Bernie's seat back and let him sleep more comfortably, and other passengers wouldn't have to climb over him. It would be easier for everyone--I hoped, and we'd be able to use the private airline lounges between flights.

I spent hours, literally, with airline reservations coordinating all our flights and arranging for wheelchairs. Our final destination was a small community in northern Germany up by the North Sea. But first we had to go to Hanover. Travel time is 17 hours from Los Angeles to Hanover. It was not something to look forward to. The hospital would pick us up at the airport, about an hour away by car. We'd be exhausted--anyway, I expected I would be. It would be really cold for us Angelinos, so I got out the warm clothes we have for our winters in France, but mostly we'd be inside anyway.

Bernie was incontinent. We had to take diapers with us--and a change of clothes and some plastic bags on the plane, just in case. Again, not something to look forward to, but there it is. If Bernie slept, if he was that sedated, I wouldn't wake him up for any meals.

The cost of surgery eliminated most of our 'rainy day reserve.' But if this wasn't a rainy day, nothing was. I didn't think anyone was getting terribly rich on this. The price, for a ten-day stay, covered *everything*. It included Dr. Goldsmith, the rest of the surgical teams, anesthesiologist, operating room, all testing, Bernie's room, and a bed and meals for me. Even if we had to stay an extra day or two, there would be no nickel and dime charges for every pill or bandage. There wouldn't be any hidden or surprise extras, it was a complete package, to be paid in advance. At our expense, Matt and Jean-François would stay in a nearby hotel.

Depending on where you live, keeping an Alzheimer's patient in a decent care facility, plus the cost of medicines and doctor visits, and an aide to dress and groom him can easily run over $60,000 a year. It is not unheard of for it to cost $5,000 a month if a patient is kept at *home* and needs 24-hour professional care--and most eventually do. Alzheimer's rips your heart out and puts you on the fast track to the poorhouse. It's an incredibly expensive disease and most people get precious little government assistance. Unless you have long-term care insurance, which we didn't, you can be wiped out in no time.

The full cost for everything would be $55,000. I was already staggered by the $43,000 a year I had to pay Royale, and that would increase annually. As Debby reminded me, I wasn't at all sure I'd be able to bring him home after surgery, but I had to give him a chance, even if it took our last dime, and like Scarlett, I'd worry about all of that tomorrow. If it came to it, I'd rent out rooms, or I'd rent the entire house and move in with a relative. I'd find a part-time job or baby-sit. I'd get a reverse mortgage, I'd sell everything, I'd borrow, I'd do *something*.

ೞೞ December 31, 1998 ೞೞ

Matt and Zeli were married today! Dano got Bernie all spiffied up and brought him to the wedding. He walked down the aisle with Matt and me, Matt guiding him, and then sat quietly during the ceremony. We had hoped to avoid giving him his meds that morning, but Hannah phoned early and said he was being difficult, so they gave him half the regular dosage. That made him somewhat sedated. He never knew where he was or why, mostly wandered aimlessly around with Dano in tow, but otherwise he was OK.

Shortly after we came home from Seattle, Matt and Zeli told me that they were going to get married in a month--so there had been a lot of busy preparation. Debby was lucky to get an airplane ticket at the last minute, so she was there, too. It was a happy day. Nineteen years ago Deb brought us Jean-François and the "French Connection." Now Matt had brought us Zeli, "The Girl from Ipanema." Life is good.

ଔଔଓଓ

Prayers and Good Wishes

Except for Debby and Matt, I didn't tell anyone what we were going to do until just before we were scheduled to leave. I didn't want to explain, to hear anything negative. It was just too hard to talk about the details, too hard to talk about it at all. But when I finally did tell, everyone I spoke to, family, friends, neighbors, even strangers, told me that they would pray for Bernie, that they would have their prayer groups pray for Bernie, and wanted to know the exact day of the surgery. People said they would be thinking of us, wishing us the best, sending their good thoughts with us--and I accepted it all, held it close, appreciated and treasured it--no matter what the source or the belief. It was all good positive energy, and God knows, we needed all we could get, that's for sure. I'd take someone's prayers to an oak tree if it would help.

Still, there were those who added little qualifications. "Don't expect too much." "Don't count on bringing him home, he'll still have to be in a facility." "Don't get your hopes too high." I vacillated about all of that myself and said that if there was no improvement, I'd be disappointed but not devastated because Bernie and I would just be in the same place where we were in the first place.

I wouldn't know until we came back home that most people, regardless of what they'd told me, thought that I was on a fool's errand.

Everything, including a planeload of prayers and good wishes going with us was in Bernie's favor. Odds were 50/50 there would be some improvement--not too bad. His health was very good, he's naturally strong, and when he wasn't medicated his mental state was--well, what's the word? Let's say his mental state was what it was for his condition. Then there was my positive Pollyanna personality--I couldn't change that--although sometimes, it annoyed even me, but there it was. So things could go well, should go well, but the risks were there, I knew that, I just didn't dwell on them. *Que sera sera.*

Now, as it happened, we'd been having some of our most beautiful picture perfect postcard Los Angeles winter days--in the high 70's. Soon we'd be near the icy North Sea. Burrrrrr! If this all worked for my sweetie pie, I thought, he was gonna owe me big time.

•NINETEEN•

January 1999

En route: Los Angeles, California to Hanover, Germany

One day, a week before we left, I called Royale Park and asked them not to give Bernie his meds that morning. From what I'd read and understood, not everyone was going to believe this surgery could help Alzheimer's and I thought it would be a good idea to film him, to show how he was beforehand.

For the video, Bernie was his usual self. Confused, garbled speech, no understanding, not knowing where he was, unable to identify a simple room key, no eye contact, ambling aimlessly about the room. True, he probably had some residual meds in him, but not enough to make him behave like that--no, it was a tragic, heart-breaking visual record of someone with severe Alzheimer's.

But something bizarre happened in flight, I'm not sure what. I'd kept my watch on Los Angeles time so that I knew when to give Bernie his meds, I didn't want to take any chances that he might become violent, but for some reason, Bernie became very rigid, his legs were like concrete pillars when we wanted him to sit down, which I'd never known him to do before. Maybe he was frightened about sitting in a wheelchair and that's why he stiffened up, perhaps it was some of his meds, or it could have been another manifestation of the disease. And although he'd been talking a little when I came to pick him up at Royale in the morning--all gibberish, of course--he didn't have anything to say once we were on our way. With the pills we gave him, I wasn't that surprised, although he wasn't fully unconscious. In fact, I had to keep my hand on his seatbelt during the entire flight. Even sedated, he kept trying to undo it and his trouser belt as well.

I wouldn't have been able to make the trip alone, especially when Matt took Bernie to the men's room. We had heavy coats and carry-ons, it really took both of us, with airline help from Los Angeles to England and from Birmingham to Hanover. All their personnel were super. Wheelchairs and assistance were always there and using the lounges made everything a lot easier.

But each time we moved Bernie from wheelchair to airplane seat then back to wheelchair his body became more and more difficult. Arriving in Hanover, a man from the hospital met us in the gangway. It took him, Matt and two other men to get Bernie out of his seat and into the wheelchair. Bernie simply would not bend his legs and arms; they all but carried him out like an ironing board. By the time we picked up our luggage, the entire airport was eerie and deserted, everyone else was long gone. It took them another good twenty minutes to get him seated in the taxi. For a while I thought we'd have to strap him ramrod straight onto the roof like a pair of skis--he would not sit and he would not speak. When we finally left the airport, dusk was falling and snow covered the countryside. We were driving through Currier & Ives.

Das Krankenhause

We arrived at Bad Pyrmont, one of the many resort spas in the area noted for its healing waters. It was essentially spared during WW II until American tanks rolled into town at the end of the war. If any of the inhabitants still harbored any Aryan attitudes, they were quickly dispelled when *schwartze Soldaten* climbed out of the tanks. By all accounts, our black soldiers were accepted and there were no reported problems on either side.

Shortly after that, 1,200 German veterans, many amputees and otherwise badly wounded, were brought to the community, placed in private homes and the families were told to take care of them. As time passed, love affairs between the veterans and the locals turned into marriages, others simply chose to stay on, and eventually the citizens built a hospital for them, and that was the beginning of *das Krankenhaus*, Bathildis, the hospital where Bernie would have his surgery.

The hospital had expanded over the decades, rooms modernized, all the latest state-of-the-art equipment in the way of CT scans, MRI's, and a monster of a machine that takes an angiogram to trace the blood flow in the brain.

A well-experienced neurosurgical team was headed by a Professor of Neurosurgery. Wholly focused on neurosurgery, he inspired confidence at a time when people needed it the most. The doctor who was Chief of Anesthesiology and Chief of Hospital Administration was also a member of the team. He looked and acted like a crewman on the rescue trucks Matt used to work with at the racetrack--rescuing is not a bad quality to have in a doctor, and his English was excellent--a big help.

In addition to these two, there was a black doctor from Africa who had studied medicine in Moscow. He was married to a German woman and they lived in this pretty little town, and I kept thinking of him as American. His English was not very good, but I directed my questions to him, expecting that we would communicate more easily in English. It probably confused him, it was just a funny trick of my brain and his non-American accent always startled me. The rest of the medical team was rounded out by handsome, young Central Casting Nordic types. There were also interns going in and out, technicians, and plenty of nursing staff--many spoke excellent English.

The hospital had done about forty omentum transpositions, half for spinal cord injuries, and half for stroke victims. Obviously, they served a much wider area than just this community. They did a tremendous number of brain surgeries and many foreigners, like us, came from all over the world. Bernie would be their second Alzheimer's patient, after the woman in Texas.

We were put in a semi-private room. I had one bed and Bernie, the other, but he kept getting out of bed, roaming around, touching everything, and going out into the hall. I couldn't control him and finally called the nurse and she found him polishing a serving cart in the corridor with the hem of his hospital gown. She put him back to bed and restrained him with a band across his middle. He could move around and sit up, but not get out of bed. He didn't say anything, didn't complain, just smiled and soon fell asleep.

The Big Day

The staff was delighted with *Herr Weiss*, which means Mr. White in German. I tried to explain that he was 100% Hungarian. They'd have none of it. They wanted him to be the German-American returning to his origins in Deutschland. I told them that, in fact, I was the German. Although born in America, my parents sometimes spoke the German they learned from their parents when they didn't want us *kinder* to understand. I added that my maiden name was the very German 'Filtzer.' They nodded knowingly to each other and declared me Hessian.

I was also told that 'Filtzer' is what they call felt tip markers, which makes sense because our family name came from ancestors who made felt hats. Now both Bernie and I were German-Americans returning to Deutschland, but at that moment, all I cared about was that they took good care of my *bohunk*.

Ben, the stroke victim we'd had lunch with in Seattle, had already had his surgery. Like Bernie, he was an engineering type and knowing that he made the decision to have the surgery on his own had helped me to confirm that I did the right thing, that Bernie would have gone along with it as well, even if he had fully understood its extent.

Early in the morning Bernie had all of his pre-op tests. By then his regular meds had mostly worn off. He was more alert and cooperative, but the angiogram was painful. He moaned a lot, but still said nothing. Matt and I stayed with him when we could, but it hurt to see his hurting. And I couldn't bear to watch them shave his head. I know it didn't hurt, but I always loved his hair, even now that it was gray, so I left the room. It was silly, but that's what I did anyway.

Because we knew that naysayers would say Bernie didn't really have Alzheimer's, I gave permission for them to take a minuscule bit of brain tissue for a biopsy. I knew that that procedure was done during other brain surgeries, it wasn't unique. The results wouldn't make any difference to Bernie and the outcome, but I understood it was important to establish that he didn't have one of the dozens of other conditions that people mistakenly call Alzheimer's.

When they took him into surgery, Dr. Goldsmith suggested that Matt and I walk in the village, there was nothing we could do sitting in the hospital for several hours. Dr. Goldsmith would release one end of the omentum, surgically elongate it, feed it up under the skin of Bernie's chest to the left side of his neck, behind his ear and lay it on the brain where the neurosurgical team will have completed a standard craniotomy. All very straightforward, just the way it's been done for stroke victims many times over.

So Matt and I walked to the village, antsy of course, but we strolled around, looked in the shops, had lunch and waited for the day to drag by. They finished just about the time we came back. The surgery went well, better than expected, and soon we were all in post-op, watching Ben continue to come around from the same procedure just the afternoon before, waiting for Bernie to do the same--and that's when it all began to fall apart.

Not Responding

I know just enough to know that all the vital signs on Bernie's bedside monitor were normal, functioning well. Blood pressure, heart, everything was fine, but it bothered me that he didn't wake up. When his eyes would open, I'd see too much of the whites. The irises moved around and rolled back. It frightened me, but there didn't seem to be anything wrong.

I was reminded of how the meds did such a number on him when he had colon surgery a few years before, but I didn't remember this sort of reaction. Of course, his disease was much further along now, but I was uneasy and so was Matt.

Matt and I realized people were looking for Bernie to be the Poster Boy for this surgery and its chance to help other Alzheimer patients. I knew that early on and I was certainly not opposed to it, but I wanted the operation for him, and if it benefited others in the long run, well, so much the better. But I didn't want people to hang too many of their hopes on him. I just wanted to alleviate some of his suffering from Alzheimer's, to keep him from having to be sedated all the time.

No reputable doctor wants to lose a patient, or to leave him worse off than he was before treatment, but I thought these doctors had the added dimension of watching how Bernie reacted in a more dispassionate way than I did. We all wanted the best for him, but for different reasons, and I was not familiar enough with all of this to know if his responses were normal. He was only their second Alzheimer's patient, so they might not know exactly what to expect either.

When they do the same surgery for stroke patients like Ben, they have a patient fully aware of what's going on, someone who is anxious to get up and get going on with life, but Bernie didn't have that same outlook. God knows what he was thinking--if he was even thinking at all.

Because he wouldn't rouse and cough, they used some sort of thumping device on his back to keep his lungs clear to avoid pneumonia. It was all very weird, he wouldn't respond the way Ben did, there was no change, but on the third day, they brought him back to our room anyway. I was not happy about that, I didn't want to be responsible for watching him, but they said he'll be OK. That's what they kept telling me--he'll be OK. His head was still bandaged, but I'd seen Ben's zipper scar across the top of his head, just like Frankenstein's creation.

At night I couldn't sleep in the same room with him. There was so much gurgling going on from his inability to get the phlegm up from his throat that I finally took a blanket and pillow to bed down in the visitors' lounge. I knew the nurses would check him on their rounds; I was wholly exhausted from lack of sleep.

As planned, Matt went home three days after surgery. He'd have stayed if I wanted him to, but I preferred that he leave, it was better for me in a way, and there was nothing he could do for Bernie who had to wake up soon, that was for sure.

But Bernie was not waking up. He responded when his feet were tickled, when they pressured the quick of his fingernails, but only with moans, no words came out. If that's the case, he couldn't be in a coma--but to me he seemed comatose. Was it still meds from the surgery? Although he was reacting to stimulation, he couldn't be awakened, and I began to stop eating. If I got even one bite of food in my stomach, I felt sick.

Finally his eyes stopped rolling around, but they still frightened me. His hazel eyes had always gone from yellow, to blue, to grey, to green. But now they became a strange cold slate apple green that I'd never seen before, and without any of the normal brown flecks in them. How could that be, could it be the drugs that they'd change color like that? And he had tiny pinhead black pupils that saw nothing. It was scary. His eyes were dead.

By the fourth day, even Dr. Goldsmith was concerned. I thought he wasn't sleeping nights either. News that Brian Sternberg, the pole vaulter from Seattle, was now standing in his metal frame for several hours cheered him, but he was clearly concerned about Bernie. They took another MRI and it showed everything was normal.

A doctor gave Bernie some sort of shot and said he should awake briefly in a couple of minutes. Amazingly, he did. He was quite alert and responsive, but only for another few minutes and the doctor declared again, "It'll be OK." I believed him, I had to. If something was really wrong, even the shot, whatever it was, wouldn't rouse him, would it?

I asked Bernie, "Do you love me?" I didn't know if I was heartened or not when he returned a very weak nod, but said nothing. He hadn't said a word since we left Los Angeles, not even gibberish, and what was all that extra, intense rigidity about? Could he have been overmedicated from Royale and what I gave him in flight? But I never gave him too much, I was certain. I know I didn't give him more than he normally took, and I hadn't given him anything for about fifty hours before surgery began. He'd been alert during his pre-ops.

The doctors kept asking me how he responded at Royale, but I told them I wasn't always there, and besides, it wouldn't be an accurate picture because he was always sedated. I didn't see how we could compare. As time went on, I realized more and more that I really didn't know his true condition when I decided to have the surgery. I was only seeing him once a week or so, and I never thought to ask anyone at Royale how he was doing because it was obvious to me that he was failing rapidly. I didn't know about the manifestations he was displaying now. I never told Dr. Goldsmith and the others about them because I hadn't seen them.

Now I began to think that he was much more advanced before the surgery than I thought he was. But one thing I did know--the man I left Los Angeles with was not the man I arrived with in Germany.

♦TWENTY♦

Rita Hayworth

It was a time when glamour was really glamour, and Rita Hayworth was fabulous. She was born to play *"Gilda."* men all over the world fantasized about her; she married a prince and gave birth to a princess. Teen-aged girls spent hours in front of mirrors trying to be just like her. Then her life just went into the dumpster. She became an alcoholic, it was common knowledge, even though her daughter, Princess Jasmine, kept saying that wasn't true, that she was sick with some sort of brain disease. But everyone knew she was drinking because of the failed marriages, the failing career, aging, you know how Hollywood types are.

And then there was the time she got off an airplane in Europe, drunk as a skunk, and they tried to say she wasn't. But pictures don't lie; at least they didn't back then, or did they?

Finally we all learned that Rita Hayworth really did have a weird disease that no one could pronounce, and that this lovely, lovely woman suffered with it for many years until she died, sometime in the late 1980's, and not that old. If it's difficult for those of us coping with

Alzheimer's today, imagine how it must have been for those when the awareness was just beginning. Belatedly, I pay them tribute.

This history all came back to me because I had this sense that 'something' happens on an airplane to Alzheimer's patients, that something happened to Rita Hayworth and to Bernie as well.

I always knew that Bernie was worse when he was in a strange place but after six months he had become well acclimated to Royale. Then one morning I took him away. I moved him in cars, vans, and airplanes, up and down elevators, crossed time zones to another continent, another hemisphere, gave him jet lag, then put him to bed in a strange building with strange people whose language he couldn't possibly understand. No wonder there was a decline.

I also came to realize that the worst change in Bernie's odd behavior came in Paris, back in 1993 after we'd taken that trans-Atlantic flight to visit Debby. Then there's the idea that light affects our brains. You know, chickens lay eggs at sunrise, and now I messed up Bernie's entire circadian clock. Plus, in an airplane, there's the change in altitude with less oxygen, adjusting cabin pressure, noise, constant droning, vibration, and bumping around. It wasn't surprising then that that horrid monster Alzheimer's began to consume him like gangbusters--we had messed up his entire comfy zone pretty bad--and he wasn't happy about it. Well, *tant pis*.

Still, I was concerned. I knew that the doctors conferred about Bernie in a little knot outside our door. They'd see him each day as a group, and sometimes one would come alone. I knew they were watching him, but still----

Improving?

Bernie seemed to improve. He grabbed the side-bars, lifted his arms high, and moved his legs on command, but he still stared off into space. I kept trying to feed him but with little success. Eventually I got a few bites of a banana in him and he passed some gas. When he did, he looked at me and smiled, the same smile a little boy gives when he does that. So he was aware.

Later, when he soiled the bed, three nurses came in to change it and I told them it was from the banana. Only one nurse knew that he'd eaten any banana, and the other two just looked blank. I don't know why I bothered with the language barrier, but I kept trying to explain that it was the banana. Then the one nurse began translating, and they burst out laughing, and when she told me why they were laughing, a man's banana, you know, I started laughing, too, and soon we were all doubled over like schoolgirls and it just felt so good to laugh.

It was astonishing to me how someone who barely swallowed air could manufacture so much piss and poop but the nurses didn't seem to mind. They all had such a good nature, laughing and joking with each other and showing real kindness and gentleness toward Bernie. Sometimes I'd see exasperation but never a flicker of resentment at what they had to do.

But Bernie wouldn't eat. He wouldn't chew or swallow, so a staff therapist showed me how to teach him, or more rightly, force him to swallow. But it wasn't working. He clenched his teeth like the gates of Fort Knox, and I couldn't get any food inside. If I did get a dribble in, he'd spit it out. If I held his mouth shut and forced him to swallow, it took forever. I couldn't get enough in him to be sufficient. He pushed my arm away when I offered him food. He was starting to make a fist and showing anger. I worried that he might hurl that fist, although I thought he's too weak to hurt anyone--and then I realized something, something that filled me with horror.

It was the same syndrome displayed by the Alzheimer's patient, Joseph, who was dying in the home where we stayed when I took Bernie for oxygen and chelation. After his hip surgery, he refused to speak or eat. You couldn't get a morsel in him no matter how you tried. He pushed away anyone with food, showing intense hostility, swinging his fist, and then he died, simply chose to die--or so it seemed to me, unless it was the disease, I never knew. Until then, I thought Bernie had been eating well at Royale, so what was happening? And I couldn't forget that he had talked about suicide several times. What I was seeing, what I was thinking, really frightened me.

I told Dr. Goldsmith about it, he'd been beside himself. He looked terrible and I was sure he was still not sleeping. The surgery went well, there was nothing more he could do and he felt helpless, I knew that. He'd never had a patient do this. His hundreds of patients for stroke or spinal cord injuries were well aware of what was happening. They didn't have Alzheimer's. Like Ben, they were eager to wake up, to start getting better. It was different for Bernie, and apparently his other two Alzheimer's patients hadn't done this either.

Once or twice a day the DeCarlo's stopped by. They brought me fruit from the grocery, or anything else I asked for. I never left the hospital. They tried to talk to Bernie but got no response. I had no idea what they were thinking, but Ben was doing remarkably well. He was quickly gaining back his strength. They'd go to restaurants for dinner, walk about the village--all in sad contrast to Bernie--who had had the exact same surgery.

I almost felt sorry for Dr. Goldsmith, he hovered over Bernie to entice him with a fresh banana, trying to get a spoonful of yogurt into him, but nothing worked. I thought Bernie was aware enough to know, at least subconsciously, what he was doing. I was convinced he was choosing to die.

But there was more. He frequently got a very surprised expression on his face. People thought it was recognition, but I knew it was some sort of tic. He was also twitching a lot, still picking at shadows, and staring off into space. His left hand was palsied, his right arm seemed even weaker, he was moving OK, but it scared me, although it could have been nothing more than after surgery weakness. Or it could have been the drugs staying in his system for so long.

Also, I worried about his brain. I knew that the brain was not supposed to be penetrated, but what about the tissue sample for the biopsy? The omentum was just laid on the left side of the brain, like you place your hand flat on a table, but that was still 'touching.' It had to have some sort of effect. The brain must have been thinking, "Oh, oh, what was that?" So was it all just weakness, reaction to drugs, touching the brain, the evil Alzheimer's still assaulting him? How soon would it take for the omentum to challenge the Alzheimer's? Were we too late? How did I know? I just knew that I didn't like any of it. Supposing he stays like this, just a nothing with tics and no responses, just a blank stare that goes right past you. God, what'll we do?

By day seven, no matter what his condition was, I thought he should get out of bed. A couple nurses came to stand him up, but his knees buckled. The therapist came in to exercise his legs and arms--at least it was something. But mostly there was nothing until the night there was singing in the corridor and he showed signs of having heard something.

A church choir was singing hymns. I asked them to come into our room, hoping he would show some sort of further response, but when they came in and sang, he only stared blankly, never a sign of anything. Afterwards, a few who spoke English stopped to say a word or two--then they left.

When the door closed behind them, I let down his sidebar and crawled into bed beside him, holding him. He closed his eyes and I thought it was a sign of familiar contentment, but then he immediately opened them and I saw only that cold, blank green stare, nothing more, so I laid there and let my silent tears fall between us.

Day 8

Bernie slept all day with no sign of improvement. I didn't think that he was going to make it and obviously we wouldn't be able to go home as planned in two days. Dr. Goldsmith, set to go home the same time that we were going to leave, said he would stay on as long as Bernie needed him. But Bernie's wasn't going to make it; I knew that, even if the doctors didn't.

No one knew what happened. Hundreds of these surgeries have been done, and no one has ever been unresponsive like this before. Maybe it was just more advancement of the disease in those few weeks before surgery. Alzheimer's was taking over; it was just the progress of the disease, not the surgery at all. That's what I came to believe, we did the surgery too late, just those few weeks made the difference. The rigidity, the refusal to speak and to eat, being spacey, they were all classic Alzheimer's symptoms, and combined with the drugs, it was just too much. I was going to lose him, it was all for nothing.

Matt and Debby were on the phone once or twice each day, trying to get our airplane tickets changed. I didn't know what to tell them. I couldn't take him back to Royale Park, they don't have nursing facilities and besides I really wanted him home. Matt was going to get a hospital bed.

Bernie's blood count was low and he needed a transfusion. I told them that I wanted to give the blood. On top of everything else I didn't want HIV, hepatitis, or anything else. But they said 'no,' and Dr. Goldsmith assured me that the German blood supply is among the cleanest in the world--but who can be sure? I had to sign a paper to authorize the transfusion and acknowledge that it may have HIV--some assurance! That's just great, isn't it? But I couldn't let him die, so I signed. At his age, even if he gets something, it would probably be years before it showed up or caused problems anyway. They gave him three units. He seemed to look better--if that meant anything.

I was really wrong about one thing though. I remembered saying that if the surgery didn't work, I'd be disappointed but not devastated. But I was devastated--completely. A light had gone out of my life. Dr. Goldsmith seemed devastated, too. He'd never lost a patient to surgery. He's a good man, but he'll have other patients. Where was there ever going to be another Bernie for me? Even with Alzheimer's, who will ever have that smile just for me?

A Typical Day

The physicians made their daily rounds, they didn't seem terribly concerned. They asked me a lot of questions about his reactions, chatted among themselves, then left.

It was a break for me whenever a nurse or doctor came in. Unlike hospitals at home, all the doors were kept closed and the nurses' station was not out in the open. Outside our room it was as empty, quiet and impersonal as a hotel corridor. There was no hustle and bustle, no one to see or hear. No stimulation. When I told the nurses about our open hospital doors, they were aghast, but I think it's better. There, alone, I was a cloistered nun.

Other patients had visitors, behind their closed doors, of course. But it was just the two of us, literally shut away in this room, with only CNN to watch in English. Debby mailed me some English books from France--I read, did my needlework and crossword puzzles. I was picking up some German, remembering a lot of what my parents said, surprised at how much I understood. When asked, I also corrected the staff's English and answered questions about America. They could not understand why an American would come to their little corner of the world when our country had the best medicine in the world. Go explain.

Ben and Cindy continued to stop by, which I appreciated. Having them there was a support. I'd have been crazy otherwise. Ben was a wonder, so healthy and strong already while Bernie stayed the same, we were just there, and he never spoke. Not that he'd make any sense, but still not a single word.

Dr. Goldsmith ordered a blood test and it showed that Bernie was beginning to starve. I didn't know how they could tell that, but I wasn't surprised. Like Joseph, he simply would not, absolutely would not eat. I didn't know enough about Alzheimer's to know for sure if it was the disease making him starve or not, but any normal person would have eaten. Unlike poor Joseph though, we couldn't let Bernie starve at this point, so Dr. Goldsmith intervened and inserted a nasal tube to force-feed him. Alzheimer's was not about to give up so easily and neither was the doctor. I had to leave the room, I couldn't stand to see him hurt any more, although I was told it doesn't hurt, and I knew he needed calories, the IV wasn't enough to sustain him.

No! No! No!

The staff doctors kept telling me that Bernie would be alright. I wanted to feel confidence in what they were saying, but I didn't. I was beside myself. They assured me that I would be able to feed him through the nasal tube, people live that way for years and years, which is one of the things I was afraid of. I didn't want to hear that. I kept saying that I didn't know what I'd do, but a doctor told me that all I had to do was put ordinary food in a blender, put it in the plunger, attach it to the tube and feed him! Yeah, right! Or, he said, buy adult supplements and feed him that--just read the label instructions and mix it up. I knew he meant well, but I wanted to throttle him. I didn't need instructions on how to follow directions on some stupid label!

Besides, I wasn't being honest with him. What bothered me was not the doing--I could do it--but for how long, because I knew that Bernie wasn't going to come out of this. So once the tube was in, how long do I keep it there, how long do I keep him artificially alive? How long do I wait to see if and when he'll ever show signs of improvement? I tell them again, I just don't know what to do. But, no, I didn't tell them what I was really thinking, what really bothered me. The words wouldn't come out. I didn't even try.

I explained to Debby one day that I didn't know what to do. She immediately understood and echoed my unspoken thoughts back to me. "You don't know how long to do it, do you? You don't know when or how you can stop." And now, for the first time, I understood why Joseph, the man who was dying in the house when Bernie was having his chelation, was left in peace.

It was all my own doing, of course, that I didn't have a doctor at home for him, to monitor him, who knew about the surgery. For all the research I did, why did I neglect that? Dr. Goldsmith told me to take him to his doctor, but I didn't, and I didn't say anything and I knew why. I didn't want to have to explain it, to hear someone refuse to listen, to give me a hard time, and since we were between doctors anyway, I just left it at that. It was incredibly, dangerously foolish, but that's what I did.

The doctors came back, talking among themselves. They preferred that patients make return flights with their surgical staples intact. But there was no doctor to take out Bernie's staples once we were home.

Are you people CRAZY? Surely I misunderstood. Maybe you send your own people off like this, but I'm staying right here until things are all settled. I had a mental picture of myself getting on an airplane for seventeen hours with a plunger full of mashed carrots, a bizarre incontinent man held together with staples, and I thought not! NOT! NOT!

I was suddenly tired of the whole thing and could not, absolutely could not, think of anything else to say to anyone. I moved to my bed, curled up in a ball, my back to the room and everyone in it. The most peaceful tranquility came over me. I don't ever remember feeling that way before, floating, not a single thought in my head, just complete tranquility. Someone was taking my blood pressure, but I just laid there. Who cares? Nothing mattered but the tranquility.

A Turnaround

There was no question in my mind that without the nasal feeding tube Bernie would have willed himself to starve, and I wouldn't have blamed him in the least, or else it was the Alzheimer's doing its dastardly deeds.

But I wasn't willing to let him go when we were so far from home. Neither were Dr. Goldsmith and the others. He was just too healthy, like it or not, and he'd been through too much to let the possibility of improvement die with him. In spite of my seemingly hysterical thoughts, I was really OK. I never screamed or yelled or fainted or accused anyone. My blood pressure held stable. I knew they were trying, Bernie was getting excellent care, and I was just stressed out from years of coping and now this, alone in a foreign country among strangers, dependent on them for everything and not always understanding their language and their ways.

Ironically, Bernie was the only one I could really talk to, so I decided it was time I had a 'conversation' with him, one-way, of course. Alone in our room, sitting on his bed, I told him that I wasn't going to let him go, that I loved him, that we still had a lot to do. I wanted him home with me, promised that we'd go home, and have all sorts of wonderful times together--get his favorite waffle with strawberries at the coffee shop, things like that. He kept drifting in and out of awareness, but I thought the feeding tube was giving him strength, and that my words might be getting through. He wouldn't leave me, he never did before, things would work out.

As usual, Matt phoned that morning, and as I often did, I put the phone to Bernie's ear. I could hear Matt ask him if he wanted to work together on fixing up our Nomad, and then Bernie, faintly, said, 'Yeah.' His male nurse was standing nearby and grabbed me when I cried out, "He spoke, he spoke, Matt, did you hear, he spoke?" The nurse was normally very reserved, would never have touched me, so I knew he, too, was deeply moved when Bernie finally said his first word in well over a week. I think he thought that I was going to swoon, he was sort of holding me up, but I was OK. Excited, but OK.

After that, lots of little things happened. He raised his legs without being asked when they were putting on his hospital stockings; he stiffened his upper lip like men do when he was being shaved, things like that. He was much more alert, and I think he liked being fussed over, especially being shaved. The drugs were finally leaving his system and the omentum must have been working already. He was making normal eye contact, sometimes responding normally to voices and TV, indicated when he'd had enough of the repetitive CNN and wanted it turned off. He hadn't done any of that in months! Of course, it could all be related to his not being drugged any more, but I remembered just why it was we gave him drugs in the first place, so everything was not all that clear-cut.

But he still had that common Alzheimer's fear of water, resisted letting the nurses wash his arms and legs, got a steel grip on the sidebars, cried out, 'no, no, no,' and winched when they give him a back rub. I've known of people who won't bathe when they get old and sick. I didn't know if they had this problem with him at Royale. No one ever said so, but it was quite possible.

They'd also taken out his internal catheter and were using a condom catheter now. I couldn't blame him when he resisted that. Too often it just slipped off anyway.

He was also walking, somewhat. The first time he had the same delighted smile a baby gets when taking his first steps, and he smiled each time he walked further and further, but it was not very far, only a matter of yards. The stiff legs and the Alzheimer's shuffle were gone. Allowed to hang loose, his arms moved normally at his sides.

When we walked out into the corridor, he became aware, for the first time, that he was in a hospital. He was still pretty rubber-legged, needed support, and was so skinny. With his shoes on, he had Minnie Mouse legs.

Almost moment to moment he was getting physically stronger, more mentally alert, said a few more mumbled words, nothing sensible. But, oh my, he still had miles to go, and his progress was glacier-paced.

The best part so far, the very best part is that that horrible Alzheimer's 'stoop' was gone. I hadn't seen it since he first sat up after surgery. As weak as he was walking just a few steps, he walked with his head held high and erect. What a sweetheart! Don't you just love it?

But They Were Right!

So the doctors were right. I finally knew that he was really going to be OK. So did I worry for nothing? No, of course not. I worried because I loved Bernie and I couldn't bear to see him the way that he was. It was just the drugs from surgery, the Alzheimer's, and the plane travel working on him. I wasn't prepared for it and that made it all so scary, maybe I overreacted in my ignorance. I didn't know if the German doctors had ever seen quite that reaction either. I never asked, they never said.

Physically he was fine from the surgery; there was never any problem with that. Thinking back and recalling what the counselor told me at UCLA about Alzheimer's patients who have surgery, and remembering the horror of his behavior when he had colon surgery, I should have been more aware, but I wasn't.

None of the medical people I dealt with when Bernie had his colon surgery prepared me in advance. No matter which specialty, which school, which country, dealing with dementia should be as much a part of medical training as learning about allergies and other pre-existing conditions that may affect the outcome of any procedure, and the family must be made aware of the possibility of abnormal reactions from Alzheimer's patients.

One of the doctors came by one afternoon and Bernie recognized him, a very good sign. He told Bernie that everyone was watching his progress, that he could become the 'breakthrough' case, maybe even be on TV. It made no impression on Bernie. Again I was reminded that he was more than just another patient to several doctors, and while that was all terribly exciting, at that point, all I wanted to do was get him home and start building him back up. Bernie did wake up long enough one night to pull out his nasal tube, another good sign.

He had to be spoon fed and fell asleep after every one or two bites, but one day we had our lunch trays in the visitors' lounge. We sat by the window and watched the blustery weather--or at least I did. Bernie had no idea where we were and kept dozing off anyway.

Between dozing, he would stare at a calendar on the wall, so I took it down and let him look more closely at the pictures. One showed a party scene with a young man and a pretty woman whispering together in a corner. I asked Bernie if he knew what the man wanted from the woman. He rolled his eyes knowingly and got a sly smile on his face, so you see, there's still some life in the old boy--somewhere.

He finally shook hands with Dr. Goldsmith when offered, although if he knew what he did to him, he might not have been so friendly. Until then, he'd shown him a fist when he came by. I could see that Bernie was worried, that he had a lot of questions, but he couldn't hold his thoughts long enough to verbalize anything that made sense.

He called me 'honey' and had more intimate expressions for me, winks and such, but I didn't know if he really knew who I was because he'd begun to flirt with all the nurses. He should only know that with his no longer bandaged, zipper-designed bald head, chicken-boned body, and white hospital drapery, he looked just like Mahatma Gandhi. Some charmer! But I'll keep him.

Doctors had been asking him over and over if he knew his wife's name, and finally, after many days and much prodding, he barely said, 'Betty,' and it pleased them no end. All his vital signs were excellent. Thankfully, he didn't appear to have a thing wrong.

But I could see that he was really frightened, and still ate far too little. He was too weak to hold his own fork, so I fed him. After each bite of food, I had to physically force him to swallow the way the therapist showed me, or shout, 'swallow' to remind him; and because he kept falling asleep, I had to shout, 'Bernie.' He'd wake with a start, open his mouth, swallow when

I commanded, then fall asleep again, although he was staying awake longer for the most part. Sometimes my yelling annoyed him, and he'd say 'Don't do that.' I considered those few words at the appropriate moment to be a great improvement. The German hospital staff will never forget the English word 'swallow,' or the name 'Bernie,' since I yelled it all day long.

The DeCarlo's left for home. They seemed so full of vitality that I had a vision of their dancing all the way to the Hanover Airport. I was now even more alone, but that was OK, I knew it was only for a few days, and I kept seeing more improvements.

One night, when I turned on the bathroom light, it shone in Bernie's eyes. He covered them with his right hand and said 'Wow.' I had turned it on every night, but that was the first time he reacted to light and it was all in the right way, even though doctors had been shining flashlights in his eyes every day with no response.

It was Day 12, and I felt that I had personally passed through my own Marathon wall, that I could go on now. I just hated feeling so little control and so abandoned. But I was beginning to feel like my old self, and anxious to get us home.

•TWENTY-ONE•

January 27, 1999

"The statistics on sanity are that one out of every four Americans is suffering from some form of mental illness. Think of your three best friends. If they are okay, then it's you."

Rita Mae Brown

We were supposed to leave on the 27th, three days past our scheduled departure date. There was no problem with our staying extra days for Bernie to gain strength for the flight and no extra charge. That was always the deal, a ten-day stay or whatever it took, and that's the way it turned out. As an American, used to paying for every aspirin and bandage, I was pretty impressed.

They finally took out Bernie's staples--dozens of them across his head, abdomen, chest and neck. And, yes, I left the room when they did that, too.

We were going to be picked up about 4:00 a.m. We had to be at the Hanover Airport by 6:00 a.m., to get our tickets changed for London. Deb and Matt had been on the phone for days getting everything re-arranged with the airlines. They were waiving the normal penalties for changing our flights and would have wheelchairs waiting for us at every point. All I had to do was go to the front counter since it was all taken care of.

Because of our staying extra days, Jean-François would meet us at our airline counter in London's Heathrow Airport. It's only about an hour and fifteen-minute flight from Hanover, so with the ambulance driver's helping us to the plane and then help from the airline, we'd be OK for that short hop. I could hardly wait.

"Zhoh"

'Zhoh,' that's the way the Germans say 'so' and they use it in exactly the same way, *zhoh*. *Zhoh*, that's taken care of, *zhoh,* we can go on now. And *zhoh*, finally, it was time for us to go back home.

The nurse came in at 3:30 a.m. I hadn't slept more than a troubled hour, I was just too excited. Breakfast and a snack for the flight were brought to us. Bernie had been given something to prevent any bowel movements on the way home and the nurse showed me how to put on the condom catheter. Then she taped a urine bag to the stocking on his leg. I was glad it was on the stocking and not going to pull the hair on his shin. She assured me that the bag would hold enough urine for the flight home because there was no way to empty it. My carry-on bag was filled with diapers, extra condoms and bed protectors which I planned to put on the airplane seats, just in case. And I had the hospital's letter saying that it was OK for Bernie to fly. I couldn't imagine why I needed that, but I took it anyway.

I was all packed, and wearing my old purple traveling sweats. The new suitcase I just bought had a broken zipper, but the nurse taped it with medical tape, so it would hold. I fed Bernie and decided to eat a yogurt. I was immediately sorry and felt sick. I hadn't eaten in days. My stomach was churning like a cement mixer but the driver arrived and I didn't want to take time to use the bathroom--I could wait until I got to the airport.

"Things Are Getting Curiouser And Curiouser."

'Alice'
"Alice in Wonderland"

We left as we arrived, in a light snow, the night air pitch black. Bernie, wonderfully aware and wide-awake, was bundled in the front seat next to the driver and I was in back clutching our passports and tickets. We had plenty of time to get to the Hanover *Flughafen*, and since Debby and Matt had everything arranged with the airlines, how was I to know that we were already sliding down a rabbit hole into *Wunderland?*

Driving through sleeping villages, quiet towns, on the *autobahn* and along country roads, I had no idea where we were, although I could read some of the directional signs we passed, so I was confident we were OK. Then suddenly the driver stopped in the front yard of a darkened building, turned on the car's interior lights, took the keys, said something terse in German, loped off into total darkness and left us sitting there!

Gott in Himmel, the man can't be such a *dummkopf* that he thinks he can get away with setting us up! After all, everyone knows where we are and who we're with, don't they? Maybe he just went to relieve himself, but then why was he running off?

All I could think about was protecting Bernie's head and holding onto our passports. I kept telling myself nothing bad could happen, it just couldn't, could it? It seemed like forever when a dark car without lights drove up and stopped next to us. Oh, God! But the car's driver was our driver. He got back into our car, told me something I couldn't possibly understand, and we drove off. Don't even ask!

After that, there was a lot of muttering from the driver and I thought he was lost. Looking at my watch, it was getting late. Oh, great! We won't get to the airport by 6:00 a.m., and sure enough, when we pulled in, it was after 6:15. He stopped in front of a building and indicated that I should get out, but I didn't see any sign for our airline. I kept asking and he kept indicating to get out.

Finally I did, but I hated leaving Bernie. I ran inside the building looking for the closest car rental booth where I knew someone would speak English. I asked for my airline terminal and was told it was two buildings down, so I rushed outside, back into the car and indicated to the *dummkopf* that he should go forward two buildings. He just sat and waved his arm ahead, as if it wasn't far and I should walk. I was gonna kill him, that's it. I'd spend the rest of my life in a German prison, but I was gonna kill him, or at the very least, perform brain surgery on him if I could only find an ax!

He wouldn't move, and I wouldn't get out. There was all sorts of construction work going on, but the road ahead was passable. I still didn't see my airline and I raised my voice. A man was walking down the sidewalk, and after thirteen years of volunteering at Los Angeles International Airport (LAX), I could spot an airport employee. I jumped out and demanded that he talk to me, I knew he spoke English. "Where's my airline?" Two buildings up he indicated. "Why won't the driver take us there? You have to ask him, why won't he take us there?" The man said something to the driver in German, I got back in the car, the man left and the *dummkopf* drove to the edge of the next building, but not past it and not to the second building. I was gonna kill him, I tell you I would, I was gonna kill him! Unlike in the hospital, I was screaming now! I screamed and I screamed, I flailed my arms, and finally, finally, grudgingly he drove to the second building and I saw my airline. One of us was not going to live to see the dawn!

Instead of helping me into the building, he sat in the driver's seat, not even opening a door. What did he expect me to do? I had luggage and a man who needed a wheelchair. He was supposed to take us to the plane, that's what I was told, I couldn't possibly do it alone.

I got out again in the dark, the cold, the snow flurries, and hurried into the building up to the counter where Debby said I should go to change the tickets, but first I had to get Bernie out of the car. I told the woman I had an emergency, I needed a wheelchair and I had to catch the 7:00 a.m., plane to London. By golly, she stopped her vitally important paperwork long enough to tell me to go stand in line at the ticket counter across the concourse and ask them for a wheelchair, then disappeared behind a partition before I could say anything else.

Well, I was underwhelmed with such courtesy and concern. The line had at least fifteen people standing there checking in with luggage, and I had a half-conscious man in a car with a crazy driver in the cold and snow, and I was supposed to stand in line! I was beyond ready to kill. I was gleefully digging a mass grave for them all.

I spied the employee I'd talked to on the sidewalk before, ran over, stopped him in his tracks and told him that HE had to get me a wheelchair NOW. He wanted to hurry away, no doubt for his morning coffee, and told me to go back to the first counter and I told him--well, never mind what I told him--just know that he quickly picked up the nearest phone and within minutes two men came with a wheelchair.

Without any help from the driver who was still warming the front seat, we got Bernie into the wheelchair and, wouldn't you know, I got another *dummkopf*. Nobody can be born this stupid. They must have a school to train them! While one man was getting the luggage out of the trunk, the idiot with the wheelchair refused to move Bernie inside where it was warm. I couldn't believe it! He was actually watching and waiting for the other man to finish unloading our bags! I started shoving him and the chair, yelling 'in, in, in,' but he kept resisting me! Then my mother's words came back from my childhood, *"Es ist kalte."* You wouldn't think I'd have to tell him that it was cold! Well, would you? Finally, grudgingly and annoyed, he slowly wheeled Bernie inside.

They got me into line at the ticket counter, finally it was my turn and I gave the woman my tickets. "These tickets were for three days ago, today's the 27th." I really wanted to thank her graciously for informing me of the date, but instead I explained the situation. I told her that the tickets had been changed and asked her to look--no, it was more like I had to twist her arm--to get her to look in her computer. When she saw our names, she was annoyed that we were actually in there.

She told me that I had to go back to the front desk to get the tickets changed. I told her I've been there and they said to come here. She was mentally calling me 'liar, liar,' and dialed the front desk to prove her point. "Well," she snipped at me, "you didn't tell her about the tickets, she says you just asked for a wheelchair."

Well, I thought, "I'm so sorry I haven't read your company rules and regulations, that I don't know the correct things to say in the proper sequence to get assistance--much less that I didn't follow the first clerk behind the partition when she so summarily dismissed me even though I said that I had an emergency, and that I could have killed her, too." But I didn't speak, just stared her down.

Once again, grudgingly, because that seemed to be the only mode of movement anyone had here, she started changing the tickets, and I asked her to check our luggage through to Los Angeles, but she said she couldn't. I tried to argue, but she repeated firmly that she couldn't, then added, "You should feel grateful that we're not charging you extra for changing your flight. I could, you know." I had to nail my tongue down. "Just get me on the London flight. I don't care about the stupid luggage." Troll! Well, I was gonna kill her, too. No one would ever convict me, it was all justifiable homicide. She was only working for the flight benefits anyway. No one would even miss her. Stupid troll!

All this time Tweedledum and Tweedledee, thankfully, had stayed with Bernie in the wheelchair then took us through Security. My stomach had not stopped grinding and the added aggravation hadn't helped. I asked if I had time to use the restroom. They said yes and asked for my luggage claim tickets, they had to do something or other with them. I rushed off and when I returned, they were gone, Bernie was gone, the wheelchair was gone. There was no sign of any of them and no one I asked had any idea where they were or what I was talking about. God in Heaven, would I never get out of this crazy house? And where was Bernie?

Across the hall a flight attendant was waving frantically at me. "Hurry, hurry, your husband is already aboard." So I 'hurry, hurry,' and sure enough, there was Bernie already in his seat being fussed over. Evidently no one had enough brain power to open the restroom door and call to me that he was being boarded, just whisked him away into a void.

Finally we were settled in and--I kid you not, our flight attendant was 'Mr. Bean.' I was *not* getting off the ground in an airplane with 'Mr. Bean.' Bernie would have to be on his own. I was mentally planning to climb out the window, crawl along the wing, and leap off the end--but then 'Mr. Bean' bent over and whispered conspiratorially, "Been giving you a rough time, have they?" Relaxing, I laughed. He'd been on this run before!

"England And America Are Two Countries Separated By The Same Language."

George Bernard Shaw

Ah, the British, so cultivated, so civilized, so courteous. It was so good to be back among them. Two very fine gentlemen met us at the gangway, put Bernie in a wheelchair and took over my carry-ons. Finally, I could relax--important people were in charge with their ties and their suits and their impressive badges and their charming manners. All I had to do was make sure that I met Jean-François in front of our ticket counter and I'd be home free.

Of course, it *was* Heathrow, an airport only slightly larger than the State of Rhode Island, but I was being treated so well I wondered if someone from Hanover hadn't called ahead and told them to be wary of the crazy American lady in the purple sweats. I explained that I didn't have my baggage claim tickets to get our luggage, but they said 'never mind, you're in the computer,' and Bernie was whisked briskly ahead while I was seated on a little motor cart tooling along, passing everyone in queenly fashion. How nice it is to be treated with proper consideration. We glided down corridors, passed up people movers, rolled into elevators, around here, around there, until finally we stopped at a counter and I produced my tickets.

Yes, I was in the computer but the clerk wanted to know why I didn't check my luggage through to Los Angeles. I explained that the clerk in Hanover had 'rules' and she wouldn't do it. They told me 'you should have told her, she could have done it,' but I reiterate that I asked, I argued, but she had her 'rules.' Besides, she didn't like me, but I didn't mention that.

I was advised, "You'll have to go back and get your luggage. You can leave your husband here with us." I was thinking, 'not in this lifetime.' Bernie had fallen into a very deep sleep. If he woke up, he wouldn't see me, I couldn't take the chance. Besides, the other man with my little motor cart was gone and I didn't have any idea how to get back across Rhode Island. I told the man with Bernie in the wheelchair, "You'll have to come with me, and stay with us until I meet my son-in-law."

Now he didn't like me either. Well, he could just join the growing list. I know, 'Ugly American.' It's not that we start out that way, it's what they turn us into, although the hard truth is, the rest of the world ain't that handsome either. Grudgingly, of course, he took us back to retrieve our luggage, and we found it sitting forlornly enough all alone in a big room. We put it on a cart and while he pushed Bernie, who still hadn't opened his eyes, I pushed the cart to another faraway counter where I was told to present my tickets so the dates could be changed, and by golly, they did it properly and without any disagreeable comments. Wow! Imagine that!

Bernie's feet kept falling off the footrests and we had to frequently stop to put them back on. There should be straps to hold them in place, but there weren't. His cap was askew, he was disheveled and drooling, all slumped into himself. People were staring, making comments about it's being Hell to get old. 'But he's not even 70,' I thought and then I turned and saw him through their eyes. My God, he looked 170. He was painfully thin, it was hard for strangers to know what was holding him together, but I knew something that they didn't know. He had inner strength, he was fine, he really was, I just had to fatten him up, his hair would grow back and he'd be fine, you'll see, he was going to be just fine.

The van that I was faithfully promised to take us to our terminal was not waiting for us, and our guide, annoyed, used a phone to call for it. When it didn't arrive and it didn't arrive and it didn't arrive--I was not at all surprised. He, however, was getting angry, and mostly he was angry at me. I snickered to myself, 'welcome to the real world of modern day air travel.' Obviously he had important work to do and pushing an unconscious man across Rhode Island while listening to his crabby wife who couldn't even keep track of their luggage was not it. Like I cared.

Finally the van arrived. It was bitter cold outside and I was trying to keep Bernie's hat and coat on while our man happily handed us off to trouble someone else. We were driven and driven half way to Vermont, taken to an odd little entrance in the back of a building, where a very agreeable chap took us up in a dinky little elevator. We got out and were pushed and pushed until, somewhere near Canada, we remarkably arrived at our ticket counter! I was impressed--bewildered--but impressed. We were seated with our luggage, carry-ons, wheelchair and coats in a little roped off area and *promised* absolutely *promised* by their gatekeepers that when Jean-François arrived, he'd be told where we were. I put Bernie's feet back on the footrests.

"Perhaps Even These Things, One Day Will Be Pleasing To Remember"

Virgil, "The Aeneid"

An officious, disagreeable little man wanted me to check in our luggage. No matter how often I told him that I was waiting for someone, he'd come back and press me again. And I was really mad at Jean-François, he was well over an hour late and I was afraid to check-in. I wasn't sure I could make the trip without him, Bernie was literally unconscious, I'd never be able to handle him alone. Where was he? OK, I was going to kill him, too.

Then I saw a new horror I had to handle. Peeking out from beneath Bernie's left pant leg was the plastic tube connecting the condom to the urine bag and it was slipping out. There was urine in it. Something had come loose, and I had to act fast. I asked the pushy man if he had some tape.

"Tape?" He was bewildered.

"Tape," I repeated.

"Tape?"

"Tape."

"Tape?"

"Tape," I shouted. I was thinking that this old geezer only had eleven months left until the 21st Century, and he was still bewildered by tape!

Pointing to Bernie's leg, "See that tube, it's full of urine and about ready to fall on the floor. If I don't get some tape---"

Poof! He handed me tape just that quick. True, it was two-inch wide white tape with big red letters "BAGGAGE" printed on it, but it did the trick and held the cuff tight.

Now I had to get him to a bathroom for the disabled and I asked the little old man in charge of wheelchairs, in his official vest and official badge, where it was. Just across the hall, he directed, but I knew better. The closest thing 'just across the hall' at Heathrow is Windsor Castle, so I asked him to take us. Grudgingly, well, you knew that didn't you? grudgingly he started pushing Bernie and we suddenly found Jean-François standing on the other side of a staircase. They wouldn't let him come in because he didn't have a boarding pass, and he couldn't get a boarding pass because I had his ticket. He had no idea where we were, and of course no one at the gate told him where we were or told us that he was there, although they had *promised* they really, really had *promised.*

Nonetheless, he joined us and we kept walking and walking, then we went outside and into another building, past the candy store until we finally stopped. Here, 'just across the hall,' was the bathroom for the disabled. I asked the man to wait for us, but he said he couldn't, he has to go push wheelchairs for the passengers--like we were stowaways!

New carpeting had just been laid and because the bottom of the door had not been adjusted, it took both Jean-François and me to drag it open. Inside was a charlady who graciously stepped outside when she saw us. The bathroom was obviously a converted phone booth with no room for a wheelchair, so we had to stand Bernie up, remember he was all but unconscious, and maneuver him inside. Besides the toilet, the walls were filled with things that stuck out and poked us. Shelves, dispensers, rolls of paper and in the corner a giant trash basket. There was barely room for the three of us to stand upright. On one side was an automatic hand drier and each time one of us stepped near, it blew hot air on us and coughed, "chaagawahwah."

Not only was Bernie's diaper soaked, but the condom had come off, just as I suspected. I tried to put a fresh one on but I "chaagawahwah" couldn't because I realized that Bernie had been lying on his back when the nurse showed me how, and I couldn't manipulate things with his standing up, and besides, his legs kept sagging, pulling him down and all but taking Jean-François with him.

We got the wet diaper "chaagawahwah" in the trash, but we couldn't get the condom on. Dear God, both of us tried and each time one of us moved, or Bernie started to tip over, we'd get a face full of fresh hot air "chaagawahwah." It was insane. I was stuck bending over in a phone booth, barely able to move, my husband's naked bottom hanging out and my son-in-law trying to put a condom on him. "Chaagawahwah." I'd never be able to live this down and I promised myself that I'd never speak to Jean-François about it again, nor would I ever tell anyone--ever. I mean, that was above and beyond what any son-in-law should ever be expected to do.

We got the condom on, more or less. I thought if he sneezed it'd fall off, but it was the best we could do and finally we wiggled him into a dry diaper. We'd been in here far too long and as we struggled to push the door back over the new carpet, the gracious cleaning lady, kept from her work, threw us a glare. Now there was no one left in England who liked us. And as we hurriedly sneaked away, behind us, I heard "chaagawahwah."

OK, so I wouldn't kill Jean-François, I'd probably be beholden to him for the rest of my life. Getting back to the airline counter, I told him to just walk past Security as if he had a boarding pass, Bernie and I had ours, and we bluffed him in.

"Beware The Fury Of A Patient (Wo)man"

John Dryden, 1681

Presenting his ticket, Jean-François was told he had to pay $75 because his flight has been changed. No, I explained, we aren't going to pay anything, it's all been arranged. So then they told us they'd be considerate and only charge us $50. That roar, that sound heard 'round the world' was the breaking of the poor camel's back--they were bargaining for $25! I no longer held my tongue, no longer had any nasty thoughts inside, I just let them all out in the crowded terminal. It was the end of the line and the poor schnook behind the counter was going to get it all. I'd show him Ugly American, he ain't seen nothin' yet!

Screaming at the top of my lungs, I become aware that I was having an out-of-body experience for the first time in my life. Hovering in front of me, above my right shoulder was an apparition of myself, and she was giggling at me. Are they allowed to do that? She thought that what I was saying was so very, very amusing!

"If you don't give him his ticket right now, by tomorrow I'm going to own this company and I'll have your job!" I had no idea where those remarkable words came from, but my apparition was hysterical and I couldn't blame her. I sounded so silly and so loud, everyone was looking, but you know, I didn't care, and the apparition just laughed, especially when I told her I wouldn't even *want* to own such a stupid company with such stupid employees.

The clerk walked away and was gone for some time. When he came back he said he'd spoken to his supervisor and she was going to waive the penalty this time. I reached for the ticket but he said that he had to tell me what his supervisor said first. I didn't give a howling hoot about what his supervisor had to say, and in so many words I told him. "Just give me the ticket!" But he wouldn't, he'd been programmed, and after the same exchange three times, I realized he wouldn't give us the ticket until I listened. "OK," I shouted, "WHAT?"

"My supervisor said to tell you this is the last time they will waive the penalty and that if it happens again, you're going to have to pay. She wants you to understand that."

"Well, thank her all to Hell and back. The next time my husband has brain surgery and I have to fly with him, I'll be sure to remember your damn penalty."

Now everyone was happy, the officious man was happy because I let him load our luggage, the wheelchair man was happy because he got to push Bernie, officially this time, onto the gangway, the clerk was ecstatic because he saw I was on my way out of his life, and my apparition disappeared and was happy just because that's her nature. Bernie was still deeply asleep.

A small wheelchair was found and two men put Bernie in it, wheeled it down the aisle of the airplane and settled him into his seat. Jean-François put all our stuff overhead, we got seated, and I heaved a sigh of relief to be heading home. Unfortunately, Jean-François was seated halfway down in coach while we were in Business. I'm not sure he'd be any help at all, especially when the carts started rolling. But we were headed home and that was all that counted.

Not So Fast, Missy

Oh, she was being far too nice, the pretty little lady in her business uniform, and I didn't like the looks of the clipboard she was holding. "Some of the crew is concerned about your husband," she said, as if I believed anyone really cared at that point.

"He's fine." More official people came to talk to me, and I was informed that the Captain was worried. I told them, "He's fine, my husband is fine."

"Do you have a doctor's letter?" YES! I do. I opened my carry-on and couldn't find the letter! Diapers and condoms were flying every which way, but I couldn't find the letter! I knew I had it, that much I knew.

"Did you give it to somebody?"

"Yes," I lied.

"Who, someone at check-in?"

"Yes, I guess so, I don't remember."

True, I didn't remember. I didn't remember what I did with it, I didn't know where it was, I just remembered that I put it in my carry-on.

Another inquisitor approached. "We telephoned and no one at check-in remembers your giving them a letter. So if you didn't give it to anyone and you don't have it---"

Liar, liar, pants on fire! I just couldn't find it, they caught me in a lie they contrived and they didn't believe I had the letter. I asked them to call the hospital in Bad Pyrmont and speak to the doctor. Amazingly they did. He said it's OK for Bernie to fly. Standing at the front of the cabin like a crew member demonstrating seat belts, I announced to all the poor restless passengers watching this debacle that it was OK now, we could leave. They were relieved.

Well, no, it wasn't OK. Now the pilot came back to talk to me. He wanted the letter. "Maybe it's in another bag, tell us what your luggage looks like and we'll bring it to you and you can find it."

I wasn't going to tell them about the suitcase held together with medical tape, I'd never get it back together, but I told them about the other little bag with all our dirty laundry. They wanted to see it, they'll get to see it.

They brought the bag to where the gangway meets the airplane door and I sat on the floor with the crew all standing around looking at me like vultures anticipating a carcass. Do they practice these looks in training? This time I knew it was MY fault, I had no one to scream at. My apparition had returned, "They think you're looking for the letter, but you know it's not there don't you?"

"Yup," I silently agreed, "it's not here."

I flipped out my dirty laundry though and found a piece of paper with German typing. Of course, no one could read it, I knew it wasn't the letter, but the pilot broadcast for any German speaking person to come over. One maintenance man did, and he translated the medical details of the surgery. They realized it's not the letter. But it was close. They put my bag back in luggage, returned us to our seats, and I announced again to the other passengers that I'm sorry about everything, and I'm *not* getting off this airplane. They can't make me get off. "But you know they can," says my apparition, "even if you give them the letter, they can make you get off." I tell her to stow it. She's no longer laughing.

Oh, good grief, the pilot came back again. He was such a baby, probably younger than Debby. I'm sure he's a fine pilot, but I doubted he'd had a lot of life's experience because the sight of Bernie just scared him witless.

"I can't fly with him, if there's an emergency, I can't put down over the ice cap."

"But there won't be an emergency. His heart is strong, he doesn't need blood, and if he needed oxygen, it's right here. He's probably in better shape than half the people on board."

My apparition silently added, "Of course, he won't open his eyes, he barely mumbles, he's too weak to walk alone, he can't feed himself, move his arms or control his hands, he has a shaved zippered head under that jaunty cap, and a matching abdomen, he's incontinent and wearing a urine bag taped to his leg, but otherwise, he's just fine, right?"

"Right!"

"You'll have to get off," the pilot said. "We'll put you up in a hotel in London and off-load your luggage."

The mini-wheelchair with two men arrived and they took Bernie off while Jean-François and I meekly followed. The collected sighs from all the passengers raised the fuselage a good two feet off the tarmac and I knew darn well our luggage was not about to be off-loaded. Airlines lie all the time, too, you know, and there's no way I was going to drag Bernie to a London hotel. And why, oh why, do they use convoluted words like 'off-load'?

Maybe the boy wonder had to set his aircraft down for a sick passenger once before and didn't want to take that chance again, but whatever his reason, I didn't care, although I admit they really tried, in their way, to help me. I still didn't know where the letter was, but I'd like to take this moment to apologize to all the passengers who came into LAX forty minutes late that night and to everyone waiting for them. I'm sorry, I'm sorry, I'm really sorry. It's just the way it went--my apparition will verify that.

♦TWENTY-TWO♦

"The Purloined Letter"

Edgar Allan Poe

Soon we were in a drafty hallway surrounded by nice enough people deciding what to do with us. Someone brought Bernie a blanket and I wrapped him in that. He'd missed all the fun, hadn't once opened his eyes, but I knew he was OK. Then we were handed back to our original airline that gave us so much trouble in Hanover. Oh, no, not after all the nasty things I said about them, oh, no! We were taken to their First Class Lounge, and as I put my carry-on bag on a table, I suddenly remembered where the letter was.

I'd put it in the side zipper pocket where it would be safe and close at hand. I opened it up, showed it to the people and said, "See, I wasn't lying, I had it all the time." All that turmoil just because I'm so incredibly stupid. I'm sorry, I'm sorry.

The airline was going to fax the hospital and when they got confirmation that Bernie could fly, they'd take us on their next flight. Evidentially the letter was *not* enough. So now we sat and waited.

My apparition declared, "None of this silliness matters, does it?"

"Nope," I agreed. "The only thing that matters is that I'm taking my husband home. I'll drag him across the polar ice cap on a dog sled by myself if I have to. All I'm doing is taking him home."

The Ladies' Room

While we waited, I felt Bernie's leg above his 'BAGGAGE' ankle and the urine bag was filling up. We had to check it, it'd already been on about eight hours and I didn't know how long it would be before we got on another plane. It should hold enough, but I wasn't sure. I couldn't lift up his pants leg because of the 'BAGGAGE' tape--I dared not remove it, so his pants would have to come down. I decided it would be best to check it in the ladies' room. I didn't want to be in the men's room with the urinals.

Half guiding, half dragging, Jean-François and I got him into the ladies' room and leaned him against a wall. Jean-François scooted outside and I told him I'd call if need be, there were no women, thankfully, inside. Holding him against the wall with one hand, I undid his pants with the other and let them fall down. Sure enough, the bag was filling up, but the diaper was dry. Remarkably, the condom was still in place, but I couldn't empty the bag because it was taped to the stocking on his leg, and it was the stocking that was slipping down from the weight of the liquid, and as it filled up, it would obviously continue to slide more.

There was a valve on the bottom of the bag, so I called Jean-François and asked him to go to the very luscious buffet spread in the next room and bring back a glass, the largest one they had. Oh dear, I know I shouldn't be writing this, but it *is* what happened. He returned with a giant crystal pilsner glass, really quite lovely--if it only knew its fate. Bernie, of course, was still out of it, being pinned against the wall in his diaper and his pants down around his ankles. Kneeling in front of him, using my free hand with Jean-François to undo the bag's valve stem and let it empty into the glass, I was thinking that if a woman should come in, she'd faint dead away. If anyone reported us, we'd be arrested for a public *menage a trois.* Our defense would certainly be unique!

Jean-François quickly emptied the glass into a toilet, rinsed it and left it on the sink while I put Bernie back together. Then we slinked away, back into the waiting room and never said a word to anyone about it--and never will! Talk about First Class passengers! I'm sorry, I'm sorry, I'm sorry. I promise I'll never do such a thing again. But my apparition was giggling.

The only reason I feel compelled to relate the story now is for those who will never get to use a First Class Lounge, since they are reserved for sophisticates like us. It's an important lesson on the proper etiquette one must cultivate in such elegant surroundings. One wouldn't want to be embarrassed by tacky behavior now, would one?

In a few hours we were boarding for Los Angeles. A steward suggested that I fax Matt from the ticket counter to tell him we were on a different flight. I wrote the info for the clerk to send after our departure, but I didn't think she understood or cared.

On board, the crew couldn't have been nicer. I hardly believed they worked for the same company I'd fought with in Hanover that morning. The three of us were seated together in Business Class and the attendants offered to help me if Bernie had to use the restroom. Yea, well thanks, but I think we already have that one covered, and no, you don't want to hear about it. They brought him extra food. Now that all the excitement was over, he was finally fully awake and starving. They offered him this and they offered him that. For the first time since we left Los Angeles, he was eating constantly and kept both Jean-François and me busy, feeding him like a voracious chick in the nest.

Once I thought he'd had an 'accident' and Jean-François and I managed to drag him into the restroom. I was kneeling on the closed toilet seat at Bernie's back while Jean-François stood in front holding him up. The door wouldn't close fully but the crew was very discreet while we bounced and bumped along, keeping him propped up long enough to check him out. Thankfully he was still dry. Mile High Club? Big deal.

Otherwise, the flight was quite uneventful. Bernie stayed awake the whole time, and as we were landing, Jean-François noticed that the 'BAGGAGE' tape was coming loose. I asked one of the crew if they had any tape. All they had were taped labels from the food galley, so we patched it with one that said 'chops.'

During our descent to LAX, Bernie zonked out again. He had to be wheeled off the plane, I kept putting his feet back on the footrests, we reported our 'lost' luggage--no, of course not, no one unloaded (excuse me, 'off-loaded') our bags like the pilot said they would, and Matt wasn't there either. The fax was never sent. *Quelle surprise!*

◆TWENTY-THREE◆

January 1999

Los Angeles, California

"Oh, Auntie Em, There's No Place Like Home!!"

Dorothy
"The Wizard of Oz," 1939

Gratefully, we staggered out of the terminal into a crisp January night, piled ourselves and a sleeping Bernie into a cab and went home. Jean-François all but carried him into the house and left him on the couch in the den while we unloaded (off-loaded?) coats and carry-ons. He was like a big rag doll but soon, while leading him to bed, he opened his eyes, looked around and seemed to realize where he was--finally, again, in his own home. I could literally see spirit and strength leap into him. He grabbed the neck of my purple sweatshirt, pulled me toward him and kissed me full on the lips, something he hadn't done in a long, long time. He looked me square in the eye and said, "Ya done good."

You can make of that what you will, I'm not at all sure just what he meant, what he remembered, what he consciously knew. Briefly, I wondered if things could be working so soon. Nah! Just coincidence? Maybe.

We got him into the hospital bed and cut the now partially filled urine bag from his leg. Unbelievably he was still dry, and also once more sound asleep, so we made him as comfortable as possible and let him be.

Matt and Zeli came by. They had stocked my fridge with enough food to feed the Brazilian Army. After we ate, they left, and I went to sleep in the twin bed across from Bernie. We all slept deeply, and vaguely I was aware that Matt returned in the early morning to drive Jean-François to LAX--he went home to the Pyrenees.

Be Careful What You Wish For

I was alone on the second night with Bernie and he soiled his diaper. I had watched them in the hospital clean him up enough times so I got my plastic gloves, plastic bag, damp cloth, new diaper, and clean jammie bottoms. All that needed to be done was to do it. Bernie, however, was resisting, strongly resisting. I got his jammie bottom off, the diaper undone, but he wouldn't budge, not one itty-bitty baby, budgie budge. His mouth was set. I tried from every angle to push, pull and turn him. I cajoled, but he doubled his fist at me and I was really disappointed. The surgery, we hoped would stop that. Of course, it was too soon to tell, barely two weeks. But he would not move and that was that. I felt the strain on my back and knew, obviously, I was not doing it right. How does someone do it alone?

It was only 11:30 p.m., so I called Matt. Thankfully he came right over. Between the two of us we got it done, but it wasn't easy, even with Matt's strength.

Surprisingly I didn't mind doing it, but it was impossible alone. I'd have to work out something.

I felt bad calling on Matt, but he said he didn't mind, that Dad had changed enough of his diapers. I know people say that, but I always felt it wasn't the same thing. Now I think, maybe it really is.

Anyway, for two weeks I'd been pleading with Bernie to eat, we even had to force feed him, and now that he's eating everything in sight, I have to deal with *this* result. One should always be careful to remember what one wishes for, it might come true!

He's Not Sick

Jace, from the Philippines, came to live with us. I must have done something remarkably noble in a previous life to have him sent to me. He was a great help, taking a tremendous load off of me, and I knew then that I couldn't do it all alone anymore. I was just too tired, too old. With Jace here I could take it easy--it would be better--I wouldn't get any younger, but it would be better.

Nights with Bernie were too much for me, I had to get some sleep, so I went back to my own room. Jace then slept in the twin bed across from him--he was restless, didn't sleep the night through and soiled the bed, he needed constant attention and Jace took care of it.

In the mornings Jace changed the linens, Bernie's pj's, and cooked something for his breakfast. He also had to feed him spoonful by spoonful, bite by bite of toast, gulp by gulp of coffee. Bernie didn't have the strength to hold anything, and besides he still easily forgot what he was doing. Sometimes I'd do it, it was time consuming, but OK. He needed the nourishment. Besides caring for Bernie, Jace did the laundry, tidied the kitchen and kept busy all the time. I knew I'd have to give him some time off. No one can be on the alert and losing sleep 24/7, even if they are getting paid.

I wanted to get Bernie back into the mainstream of life as much as possible, if that could ever be. It wasn't as if he was 'sick.' It was only natural that people who visited may have thought that way, but I always left the door to his room open so he could hear our voices, the telephone, the noise of the kitchen. I thought it was stimulating, but he was really too weak to get out of bed and he didn't even try.

Often enough he defiantly turned his face to the wall. Sometimes I let him do that, other times I'd fuss until he turned around. It depended, I didn't intervene if he was angry, I did everything to keep him from being angry, but he was mad as a hornet when he did that--turned to the wall. Somewhere he was aware that something was done to him and he didn't like it. He'd burrow into the wall again and again, like he was trying to escape his world.

He was confused about getting in and out of the hospital bed. When we wanted to get him up and dressed, I had to sit hip-to-hip with him so that he couldn't lie back down, and it took all my strength to keep him in place even though he was still weak. At the same time, Jace tried to stand him up and we often needed more than one try. Getting him dressed was a real challenge and it took the two of us, but being dressed was another part of his being in the real world.

Sometimes he had to be changed from head to foot two or three times a day--and the bed, too. We put waterproof bed pads on the overstuffed furniture in the front room when he sat there, but it wasn't enough. So I took the bottom cushions to the auto upholstery shop and had them covered in clear plastic. Mostly, though, he slept the day away in bed. His incisions were healing nicely and he got a bit stronger each day.

When a visitor came by only days after we were home and said, "Hi, Bernie, it's good to see you," Bernie recognized him and replied, "It's good to be seed." We all knew he meant 'seen,' but it was just great to have him so aware so soon. What a sweetheart!

Second Thoughts

We'd been home eleven days and Bernie was certainly a lot better than he was in Germany, but I didn't know if he was as good as he was before the surgery. I kept trying to think of how he was at Matt and Zeli's wedding only five weeks before, and I thought he may have lost ground. He was definitely thinner, paler, not as verbal, even if it was only gibberish. It'd been less than a month since surgery, and I couldn't tell what was recovery from the surgery and what was Alzheimer's, which I knew still had him firmly in its grip.

So did I have second thoughts? Oh, second, twelfth, thirty-first, a hundred and ninth, of course. Why didn't I just leave well enough alone, let nature take its course? How could I put him through all of this additional suffering? What in the world is going to happen to him in the future?

As soon as he was strong enough I planned to take him back to our original family physician at our HMO. He'd need someone anyway, like we all do, for whatever medical things came along. I was sure he was in good health, physically. Even though we spoon-fed him, he ate everything with relish, stuffing it in and seeming to enjoy it, so that was all good. It bothered me, though, that he slept all the time, looked pale and cold, but sleeping a lot is what Alzheimer's victims do.

Often I thought that the surgery would not work, that he'd be on the short end of any improvement equation, that it would all have been for naught--then he'd do something that surprised me. One day he'd been particularly difficult, looked really haggard, so I put him to bed and we both napped. When I came to him later, he looked up at me and said, "You're beautiful." He hadn't said that in a long time. I asked if he really thought I was still beautiful after fifty years, and he said, "You'll always be there." I knew he meant to say 'you'll always be beautiful.' A good moment.

On the other hand, I could ask him to give me a hug, and he might do it, then he'd hug whoever else was there as well. He'd give other people the same smile, extend his arms to them the same way he did to me, so I was still never really sure just who he thought I was. I'd been trying to get him to say 'Betty' again, and once he almost got it out. But then I'd asked him if my name was 'Susie' and he'd nod 'yes.' So go figure--I couldn't, and I didn't think anyone else could either.

We also let him walk outside in the backyard while we held him. He didn't go very far, just started off with a few steps, but the fresh air was good and each time he walked a bit further. Then he walked out front to the end of the driveway. It's on a slope, but he came back up without any problem. In a few days he was able to walk as far as he had in the hospital, always increasing it, so he was regaining strength, and I hoped it was also stimulating his circulation, getting that blood through his body and into his brain.

So, yes, I had second thoughts, of course. I'd been doing pretty well living alone after I placed him at

Royale and now he was back in my daily life. So, why, I asked myself, why? Bottom line was that I simply could not abandon him, could not sacrifice his one chance at a little better life just so I'd be free to--to do--to do what? Honestly, I didn't have anything else all that important to do.

All Alone

Dr. Goldsmith phoned every few days. I could talk to him, ask him questions and he said he'd come to Los Angeles if I thought Bernie needed him. But in truth, I didn't know what he could do, any more than my surgeon could have done anything further for me after I had my appendix out. The surgery had gone well, the patient recovered, what else was there except to wait? I'm sure I would have felt better if Dr. Goldsmith had an office here, but he didn't. He had patients all over the world I assumed he kept in touch with, but I was feeling all alone in this, and it sure wasn't his fault.

Before the surgery, Dr. Goldsmith told me to talk to Bernie's doctor about it, but he really didn't have one, it was just a quirky situation at that particular moment. It came about when I moved him to Royale and was having his records transferred to a nearby HMO facility, then he was in lockdown, then back to Royale and I just never got it all together. The doctor I took him to at Royale was a general practitioner just filling in for the moment. There was one other doctor who barely knew him, only saw him a couple times to monitor his meds. I mentioned omentum transposition to her, she didn't say anything pro or con, and I never told her that I was going to have the surgery. The doctor in lockdown was not in any way to be considered Bernie's personal physician, he only saw patients confined to that mental facility. Once they left, they went back to their own doctor--which Bernie didn't have at the time.

So there really was no doctor who knew Bernie to ask about it.

I knew that Bernie was in excellent physical health, that he could survive the surgery and the plane trip, and that's what happened. I didn't know he might try not to wake up, not respond, refuse to eat or speak, and the more I thought about it, the more I thought about Joseph, the man who was going to die, when we went for chelation. It seemed like the same pattern, except that we intervened. It may have been against Bernie's wishes at the time, but it was the only decision we could have made, I was certain of that. Everything I did was to give him a chance to improve, and I knew that chance was still there, even though I had all those second thoughts.

Bernie, who was always so fastidious about his person, still feared being bathed. He fought the sponge baths in Germany, and he fought them here. I told Jace not to let him see the basin of water and that helped a little. Now that his incisions were all healing, we gave him showers, and I could hear his shouts throughout the house, echoing off the stall tiles, yelling at Jace, "Get me the hell outta here!" They may not have been the words I wanted to hear, but they were music to my ears compared to what he'd not said the past month. Then one afternoon he asked me, "Do you love me?" That was another breakthrough. Of course, I did and that's what I told him to his pleasure.

I told all of this to Dr. Goldsmith when he phoned, it pleased him, but I really couldn't say if it was the consequence of the surgery or just the fact that Bernie was now at home and no longer sedated. Besides, he also told Jace, "I love you." So, again, I didn't know if he knew me from anyone else--although I believed he did.

He had stopped trying to pick up shadows the way he did before the surgery, and that was a great joy for me, not to have to watch him do that. It always made me shiver inside. But these remarkable improvements aside, I also told the doctor that I was feeling very alone in this--I guess he got me at a bad moment. He assured me that Bernie's sometime paleness and sleeping is not unusual for the surgery he had, especially since he really didn't start his recovery for so long and said, again, that he'd come to Los Angeles if I needed him, but I was sure I'd feel better as soon as I took him back to his old primary physician at our HMO, so I told him we'd be OK.

I didn't know what I was supposed to do. I wished that there was someone nearby like the people who monitored the first patient. This was all so new for Alzheimer's, no one knew what was supposed to happen. It's not like anyone told me I should watch his progress, but I just felt the responsibility. And, actually, I didn't know if anyone other than Dr. Goldsmith really cared. They seemed to care in the hospital. In fact, when I left Germany, I felt as if I was being entrusted with the rarest of Faberge eggs.

I frequently forgot that Bernie was a research patient, of sorts, that people were waiting to see how he responded, if there was any improvement in the Alzheimer's, and I worried that the surgery came too late. I wished it had been done a year or two sooner before he was so advanced, but I didn't know about it then.

And there was another thing. Sometimes I thought I could all but see the omentum working on Bernie's brain by the expressions on his face, or when he'd put his hand to his head. It was like a pained, quizzical expression, and it appeared to take a lot out of him, although, admittedly, he was still weak from the surgery. It seemed that it would really be sapping a lot of his energy to be producing new blood vessels, or whatever was going on in there, wouldn't you think?

I just thought of Bernie as my dearest love. Sometimes I looked at him, a shadow of himself, a true wraith of a man, and I couldn't believe it. It simply could not be, not my strong, handsome, healthy, intelligent, dependable Bernie--almost anyone else I could believe, but not him. These thoughts were so sensitive in me, that when I tried to express them verbally to Matt, the words refused to come out. But I can type them.

A Red-Letter Day

It was Tuesday, February 8, Justin's twelfth birthday. The surgery in Bad Pyrmont was Thursday, January 14, less than a month earlier, and Bernie was sitting across from me at the kitchen table in front of the newspaper I'd left there. He began some gibberish, and the only word I understood was 'activism.' That's not a word someone uses in everyday conversation, gibberish or not. His hand was on the paper, and upside down I read the word 'activism.' I literally came apart at the seams--HE WAS READING! Bernie hadn't read a single word in well over a year.

Just to make sure, I looked through the paper to find a few simple words in bold type and asked him to tell me what they said. He looked, and I kept asking, and he kept looking, and finally he said, clearly, "TIME TO PLAY." That's exactly what it said. He was reading, there was no doubt about it, he was reading. My God, he was reading!

I phoned Matt and Debby and Dr. Goldsmith. I wanted to phone the world. You can't imagine what it's like unless you've seen someone lose the ability to read, but it was a miracle to me. Dr. Goldsmith said he was going to call Germany and tell them.

After that, Bernie seemed completely exhausted and we put him in his bed. I leaned over and said, "I told you that you were going to get better, didn't I?" His smile was clear and understanding when he answered, "Yes, I know that." We were actually having a 'send-message, return-reply' conversation that made sense. Then he fell asleep.

All Day

Every once in a while Bernie would say something that astonished me. Jace said he'd shown him a magazine cover and Bernie read the word 'medicine' on it, and when an announcer on TV said that the basketball score was 51-53, Bernie said, "That's close," and to me it meant his concept of numbers was there. Later he actually followed the dialogue in an old movie, making an appropriate 'ah-ha' sexy sound when one of the men tried to grab the heroine--things like that kept happening off and on all the time. You have to realize that he hadn't followed anything on TV for a year--probably more. Who keeps track of when someone stops doing something? But then he'd drift away like always, or I'd ask him something and he'd be unable to answer, to even make a sound.

Jace pointed to me and asked him who I was and he said, "Betty Lee." He also said "Betty Lee" when I asked him our daughter's name, although later he correctly said it was "Deborah Ellen." I asked if he knew who the President was, and he answered 'no.' When I told him who it was, he shrugged and said, "What do I care?" He didn't want to know what year it was, and he seemed unable to answer that he was now in his own home. So he still had a long way to go, but good grief, it was an incredible start. I wish I could have kept a camera on him all day, but he wasn't saying things all the time. Most of the time, he was still quiet, but life was coming back into his eyes, and he stayed awake more each day.

When the handyman came by, he recognized him and said, "Hi." While that was wonderful to hear he went to sleep in the middle of it all. I was just glad Jace was here to share it, to verify everything. And he still needed someone to feed him, because he'd forget he was supposed to be eating, or wasn't able to pick up the fork from time to time.

A year ago, Bernie was following me around asking me to marry him. Now when I asked if he remembered our wedding, he said 'yes.' I asked if he knew where we were married, and he said, "Vineyard Avenue." That was correct! It was the street where my parents lived, in the house where we were married 48 years ago.

Still, he had no idea he'd been away from our home for eight months, and when I asked him who lives in this house, he wasn't sure. But these little miracles were more than OK with me. I was teasing him about his being ugly, and he told Jace, "I'm the very best thing that ever happened to her." And he said it with a wink!

He still got stuck on "I think----" or "I want----." He'd get the first thought sometimes, but couldn't come up with a second one to complete what it was that he thought or wanted. But then he'd look at a fruit bowl and say, "Look at the size of those oranges!" He also became aware of his not being able to easily find the right things to say and then he'd get playful and say things like, "Whoop-de-do" or "La-de-da" or "Toot-toot." Obviously he was covering up, making things funny--he knew what he was doing. Over all there was far less gibberish, but it was often still there.

"Here Comes The Sun"

George Harrison

It'd been raining and cold out for a few days, but I wanted to get Bernie moving, to keep up some circulation, get some energy back into him, some stimulation with people and activity, so we went to the mall. Once inside, he was glowing, almost like a child seeing his first Christmas tree, and he was walking so tall, not hunched over like before.

He looked in some windows, ignored most, and read some of the store signs. Sometimes Jace or I would ask him to read something, then he'd puzzle over it and seem unable to verbalize. We stopped at his favorite Chinese stall in the food court, but he wasn't able to choose from the array of foods. At any rate, after the walk-about, he was energized, his color was better, and I was glad we did it.

Violence

I never forgot that the reason I placed Bernie was because I feared he'd become violent and put me in the hospital. And indeed, he did become violent at Royale and had to be committed, so I'd been watching him closely since we'd been home. Then one morning, for the first time, he didn't fight Jace about being in the shower, except for when he was getting his hair washed, so maybe that would pass as well. God, I hoped so.

Several times, since Germany, he'd become terribly angry and formed fists I was afraid he might throw, and once I saw a violence in his eyes that frightened me, but nothing came of it. If he had become too aggressive, I would have had to medicate him again, and then it would have all been for nothing.

Sometimes he got angry if we tried to move him. We'd tell him to put his feet outside the car door to get out, he'd say, 'OK' but keep them inside, or if we got them out, he'd pull them back in. He'd had trouble like this for years before we knew about Alzheimer's, couldn't follow exercise directions, or really dance, no sense of rhythm--maybe it was part of the onset all along.

He'd say he wanted to get out of bed or to stand up, but there were too many arms, legs and body parts that had to be moved and coordinated for him to manage, and when we'd try to help, he'd fight it. Once he simply would not get out of the car and I was afraid he'd explode. I told Jace to just let him sit there, and after I thought about it for a few minutes, I got his baseball cap and asked him to hold it in his hand. He had to relax his fist to take it, so I knew he couldn't hit us. Then, when I had changed his focus, he let us guide him out of the car without a sign of a problem.

So I'd been thinking a lot about violence. What in the world made Bernie, the most gentle of the most gentle, turn violent? Everyone knows you can take the cutest, most loving puppy and turn it into a vicious dog. You can do the same thing to some children. Too often, though, violence can visit when it's least expected, it's not always a matter of environment. Sometimes normal people just 'snap.'

Oh, sure, some people are just cussed jerks, but maybe it's a matter of brain chemistry gone awry, a lot of things we don't yet understand. Hopefully, one day in the not too distant future, a simple test will tell if someone may be prone to violence, and then body chemistry can be adjusted to prevent it. Why not?

Mortal Combat

Of all the life and death struggles, none was more significant than the one that was going on in Bernie's brain all the time. Until surgery, it was a foregone conclusion that the victor would be Alzheimer's, there was no defense against it. Even though Bernie knew something was invading his brain, any mental efforts he made to repel it were useless. He would continue to deteriorate. If Alzheimer's followed it's normal decimation of the body, he'd become more and more unaware until he would be a literal zombie, unable to do anything. One by one, his organs would shut down, and the day could come when he might well exist in a fetal position, never moving, never again to be of this world. Alzheimer's is among the cruelest and most merciless conquerors. With any luck, he'd die before any of this happened.

But the surgery, radical though it may have been, was an option. It meant a chance to bring reinforcements to the battle for Bernie's brain. No one knew if the battlefield was on an even plane, no one knew what skirmishes were playing themselves out. All we knew for sure was at the moment the omentum had established a beachhead. If nothing else, it was overcoming the violence of Alzheimer's--at least for a time. Whether or not it could hold any more of it at bay for the rest of Bernie's life was something we'd just have to wait and watch for.

We also knew that Bernie was incredibly healthy and his system could be supplying his omentum with strong reinforcements to help repel the further advances of Alzheimer's. But the omentum was only on the left side of the brain. Would its effects spread out to other sectors, and how established was Alzheimer's anyway, how entrenched and where at this juncture?

Could the omentum hold out against the possible continued pillage of Alzheimer's, and for how long?

It all sounded terribly dramatic, but in truth, that's the way I saw it, a great silent, unseen battle raging inside of Bernie's brain. I could see on his face and by his actions that it swung back and forth, the previously unchallenged onslaught of the Alzheimer's versus the surprise invasion of the omentum was obvious to me, and the Alzheimer's didn't like it one bit. Well, as I've said before, *tant pis*, as if I cared what it liked. We all had a stake in it, no matter how it turned out, no matter how long it might last. I knew it was only one battle in a mighty war, and I knew that Alzheimer's was still going to be there at the end, but it would be worth all the sacrifice if it brought him some relief.

Continent

Another thing I was hoping for was that he'd no longer be incontinent. If *that* came about, he could sleep in our bed again with me, which I dearly wanted, but I wasn't generous enough to sleep with him otherwise. The truth is, he didn't seem the least bit interested in sleeping in our bed. He seemed more than content to stay in the hospital bed, maybe it was security for him--or so I told myself.

A couple times a day, Jace would try to get him to sit on the toilet, but he wouldn't do it. He'd had a lot of accidents at Royale, was always in diapers at lockdown, lying in bed in Germany and ever since we came home. I thought he may have come to rely on the feeling of them. But he hadn't been in diapers all that long, actually, so hopefully he could regain control. And then you never know in some of these facilities whether or not a patient is really incontinent or if it's just easier and less time consuming for the staff if they keep the patients in diapers.

•TWENTY-FOUR•

Welcome Back

Bernie had been resting in the hospital bed with the bars up when he suddenly appeared in the kitchen where Jace and I were putting away groceries. We were surprised because it was the first time he'd gotten out of bed alone, and I knew it was a difficult chore for him, even with our help. It meant he was gaining strength from the surgery, and that pleased me. Then very clearly, without any verbal faltering, he said he wanted to be with the people, meaning Jace and me. I thought to myself, "Welcome back to the world, sweetie pie."

A Crazy Old Lady

I phoned Dr. Goldsmith and told him Bernie's progress, but who was going to believe me, or even Jace? Who has ever had Alzheimer's patients like this before and knew the score?

People who hadn't seen Bernie pre-surgery would say he's just an old man answering questions, maybe a little slow or confused, but what's so special about that? No one would understand the progress he'd made or, hopefully, any progress yet to come. And, I supposed, it was just as important to monitor Bernie even if there wasn't further progress, although I hoped that would not be the case.

They'd say it was just his wife making an issue over nothing, a housewife, and what does she know? She's not reliable, not a trained observer. She's probably senile, too, a crazy old lady imagining things. It's only wishful thinking on her part. Maybe he never really had Alzheimer's anyway. Dr. Goldsmith is just a charlatan, and who goes to Germany for such nonsense? What a bunch of silliness, and wasn't she so easily taken in, naïve woman, to throw away her money? That's what they'd say.

Whenever I told anyone about the surgery, they always, *always* said that they'd never heard of omentum transposition, much less anyone's reversing the ravages of Alzheimer's. I was interested because Bernie was my husband, but good grief, this was a miracle, it shouldn't be kept hidden in our little obscure house.

The problem was, there really wasn't anyone around who knew that much about how an Alzheimer's patient responds after this surgery, so in a way, it was up to me. Objectively, I found all that happened fascinating, but I'd never thought about it before, never even knew such surgery existed nor the extent to what it might help. But I couldn't help noticing, keeping track. I wasn't sure I'd be so intrigued if the patient was a stranger, but it was my Bernie and a wonderment to watch.

I could have wished that it went faster, that he was going to return to his old self--but I knew that would never be--this, and only this, is what we had.

Altered Blood Flow In Brain May Promote Alzheimer's

Tuesday, January 26, 1999
By Malcolm Ritter
The Associated Press

NEW YORK (AP) -- Rogue bits of a natural protein may promote Alzheimer's disease by disrupting the flow of blood in tiny vessels of the brain, a study suggests.

The study provides more evidence that vitamin E and other antioxidants may fight the disease, and <u>suggests that finding treatments to restore normal blood flow may also pay off.</u>

Scientists don't know what causes most cases of Alzheimer's. Many point to overproduction of natural protein fragments called amyloid-beta, which form clumps in the brains of patients. Studies show these fragments can kill brain cells.

The new work suggests amyloid-beta, or related fragments, can promote Alzheimer's in a second way: by boosting production of harmful substances called oxygen radicals, which in turn keep tiny blood vessels from delivering the right amounts of blood to brain cells.

The study is presented in the February issue of the journal Nature Neuroscience by neurologist Dr. Constantino Iadecola of the University of Minnesota with colleagues there and elsewhere.

Dr. Zaven Khachaturian, senior medical scientific adviser to the Alzheimer's Association, called the work exciting and said it reveals "a very important part of the story" of what causes the disease.

The article went on about the research done with mice, and included these conclusions:...*that might mean the vessels can't shunt more blood to brain cells...that could damage those starved cells, or at least make them more vulnerable to damage from other causes...researchers found two bits of evidence that oxygen radicals were involved in the blood vessel problem.*

Presidents

Dr. Goldsmith, now we were 'Harry' and 'Betty,' was interested in knowing how we could substantiate what Bernie was like before. I told him that there were medical records for everything. There was also my journal, but detractors would say that I made it all up.

Records from UCLA, our HMO, and all the other doctors were available, it was just a matter of gathering them together, if anyone cared to see them. He wanted to know if Bernie has been asked the standard questions about who's the President, naming three objects, yada, yada, and I told him, yes, numerous times, or if he could now name two Presidents, but I didn't know, probably not. Bernie was still very much in the clutches of Alzheimer's.

After I hung up, I asked Bernie if he could name two Presidents. He finally stumbled over 'Franklin.' I thought he meant Franklin Roosevelt, but he couldn't get it out. I tried to pump him about George (Washington) or Abraham (Lincoln), but he didn't respond. Then, he suddenly said Franklin Roosevelt, although he again stumbled over 'Roosevelt.'

I asked him if he remembered being a soldier, and he did. I asked him where he went when he was in the Army, and he said "Fort Ord," which was correct, but I expected him to say Korea, so I asked him if he knew which war he was in. He said 'no.' And then, as

I turned away, he said "Korea." *Zhoh*, your guess is as good as mine as to where those memories had been. Maybe he would have said the same things when I placed him eight months earlier, before he was sedated, but who thought to ask?

And, of course, I wish I'd been video taping his behavior all those years, but why would I have done that? I didn't know that he'd have the surgery, that we'd want to compare before and after, but anyone who has been a caregiver to Alzheimer's patients or seen them in a care facility will know what Bernie was like. It wasn't something I wanted to memorialize.

Hidden Improvements

I just knew that he was getting better. He wasn't talking to phantoms in the air, he was following a little more TV, he continued to read isolated words, and moving on to reading phrases, all in big letters, of course. He couldn't read much text because you have to remember the lines you've just read, and without short-term memory, he couldn't do that.

He wasn't as fidgety. He'd be angry and upset at times, but not violent, and he wasn't sedated. He spoke less gibberish and could have brief, one or two sentence normal verbal exchanges, but not any more than that. A phrase here and there would come out perfectly, but too much and the word confusion returned. Good grief, I told myself, it's only a month.

He resisted bathing less, although he would still cry out 'no, no.' He may or may not show aggression. Jace, who sleeps in the same room, said that he'd been restless a couple of nights, but he didn't get out of the hospital bed and roam around, nor did he undress himself during the day as he did before.

He was a long, long way from being anywhere near normal, but if I had to say for sure, I'd say that the surgery improved his mental capacity somewhat, and his social behavior tremendously. He was a different, more controlled, more all-together person than before. And, either way, I loved him so much.

Irony

The irony in all of this was that if Bernie continued to improve, the less we would be believed! Although that was never my concern. He had not shown any further signs of improvement for a bit. He held the newspaper sideways and I asked him to turn it the right way, but he didn't understand. He read a few words I pointed out, but he was not interested, and he was confused about what to call thumb or toe, hand or foot. When I finally got him to say 'thumb,' it came out 'umb.'

He still had a lot of physical recuperating to do from the surgery. He was gaining weight--we gave him canned supplements, his color was good, and he stayed awake longer. My not-so-secret fear, of course, was that he wouldn't progress any more, that he may slip back.

He was moving around the house more and more--it seemed somewhat aimlessly. He was bound to be restless, there wasn't much he could do. He made attempts to go into the backyard alone, but didn't open the screen door. I didn't know if he forgot that he wanted to go out, if he had some fear, if he didn't know how to open the door, or just changed his mind.

But a brief trip to the grocery store annoyed him. He hadn't been there for almost a year, was uncertain about it, ill at ease, obviously wanting to go home.

But each day Jace took him for a long walk, so he was getting exercise.

As he did before the surgery, he picked things up randomly as if he was going to use them, but then didn't. So far, though, he didn't do it as often, but like the sideways newspaper, it was inappropriate. When Jace set a place for him at the kitchen table, he picked up the silverware and carried it into the den. It could have been that he thought he would eat there on a TV table, but he was unable to verbalize that.

Sometimes I felt like I was watching and analyzing too much, but I saw these things, and believed they were important. Only time would tell how far this would go, and I suppose that an up-and-down progression, the nature of the disease, was to be expected. It wasn't easy being patient, though I had learned patience years ago--since Bernie has had Alzheimer's and I'd come to understand and accept its strange parameters.

After all the initial excitement since surgery, I thought that he had definitely reached a cognitive plateau, or more correctly, in my view, a behavioral stance that we could live with, things that wouldn't necessarily show up in whatever memory tests a doctor or clinician might have for him. But these improvements were important to me, improvements that made it all worthwhile. He was certainly more agreeable and pliable, in fact, I would say sometimes too pliable. I'd like to have seen a little more of the old fire in him.

Ruminations In The Squirrel Cage

Watching Bernie was like seeing a movie being run backwards. Having seen the deterioration, now I saw some of it undoing itself, and I believed on occasion he'd be thinking--or at least trying to think--wondering, "What's wrong with me?"

Most of the time he seemed as happy as one can expect given the circumstances, but there were times when I saw such deep sadness in him that it broke my heart. He knew something was wrong, I think he's always known that something was wrong. Not every minute of every day, but sometimes it came over him like an ashen shroud, and that's when I'd think about the decisions I'd made for him--for me--for us.

And I always came back to the same conclusion. Physically, he couldn't have been healthier and had survived the surgery remarkably well. His system quickly regained full function, and all his incisions healed rapidly and well. But he still had Alzheimer's. "Hee, hee," it would gloat, "I'm still here." I should have gotten his records from lockdown and posted them on the fridge to read each day, to remind myself how things were before, because now it was so much better. "Hee, hee, yourself."

I thought of Charly in *"Flowers for Algernon"* and the patients in *"Awakenings."* With experiments they got better for a little while, then sadly mentally reverted--childlike again. Was it worth it? Should they have been left alone, never given even that small lucid life? Should I have let nature have its way with Bernie? If I thought about it too much, the squirrel would never get off its wheel. But don't we *have* to do something--if not for the Bernie's of today--at least for those yet to come? I didn't feel I could wait until a cure came along, even though that's what everyone wanted. We couldn't just do nothing, and how would we ever know what works until it's been tried?

Over and over people told me how much they admired my courage, my bravery--but I didn't feel courageous and brave. I questioned my motives--I couldn't always face what they truly were, I just felt that they were mixed. Did I turn my beloved into a guinea pig, a sacrificial lamb, just to boost my own ego? I was so sure it was going to work--but I could have been wrong. Should I have left him in peace? Ah, but then I'd think back--he was *never* at peace--not for a split second.

He seemed to be more difficult in the mornings if he'd had a restless night. I hated to think of giving him a sleeping pill, so I'd wait to see what would happen. He'd usually settle down, take a nap. Physically he was looking so good, he could be so sweet and cute, especially with his baseball cap awry--I just wanted it to work so much, but I still had fears, real fears about the future. My poor, sweet love.

•TWENTY-FIVE•

March 1999

Sharing

What I was seeing was absolutely incredible. No one was going to believe it, but there it was, his Alzheimer's symptoms were reversing. Each day his personality was re-emerging. Of course, he still wasn't normal, far from it, but a handful of people who had been with us through all of this will vouch for everything that I write.

I knew it may be too soon, but I wanted to share what happened, give others the opportunity to investigate this, talk to their doctors, discuss the possibilities, so I posted a notice on an Alzheimer's caregiver message board. It was only a few lines, headed "Some Hope." I briefly outlined Bernie's condition and the articles I'd read, then waited for the onslaught of families wanting to know about it for their loved ones. But nothing happened, not one person responded, nor did I see any caregivers mention it to each other on the board.

I soon realized that no one knew who I was. It sounded like a come-on. Why should anyone believe me? Things like that show up on message boards all the time. You know, 'read about this wonderful pill,' 'send away for free 30-day supply,' whatever. If they had asked their doctors, chances were they'd been advised that it was hokum--just another scam. I probably wouldn't have responded either. Well, it was too bad, but there was nothing more I could do at the moment--message boards were obviously out. I'd have to think about how to get it into the media, I had some publicity background, but for the moment my first priority was Bernie.

Still looking around the Internet for someone to share this with I found ~Omentum Transposition~ (http://members.aol.com/phx1959/omentum.html). I had no idea who they were. It was a site for spinal cord injuries, and over the months I'd been getting a better idea of the tie-in between the brain and spinal cord injuries. I thought, how could it hurt, and sent them an introductory email telling them about Bernie and our going to Germany. They posted it on their Web site and I was glad that it was now out there where it could be found and read by everyone. Subsequently, I learned the site is a licensed physical therapy clinic, and since 1996 some of their clients have been spinal cord injury patients operated on by Dr. Goldsmith. In their experienced hands-on opinion, omentum transposition surgery had been very beneficial to many spinal cord injury patients.

I put whatever the problems had been with Dr. Goldsmith, his detractors and omentum transposition out of mind. I'd gotten what I wanted for Bernie, in fact more than I had ever counted on, and was certain that things would change once the outcome of Bernie's surgery was known with the reversing of his Alzheimer's symptoms. It turned out that I was way too overly optimistic.

The Biopsy

The biopsy of brain tissue taken during Bernie's surgery was performed at the University of Washington School of Medicine, Seattle, Washington, and showed:

> Final Neuropathological Diagnosis:
> Alzheimer's disease.
>
> Gross Description:
> About 1 cm hemi-spherical mass of white tissue, flat and shiny on one surface; cut at right angles to this surface to give 3 pieces.
>
> Microscopic Description:
> H&E, trichrome, LFB-PAS-H, congo red and immunostain for GFAP, nau N, beta-amyloid protein and tau reveal cerebral cortex with many senile plaques surrounded by reactive astrocytes.
>
> Neuropathology Number: Np26459.

"Don't Worry, Be Happy!"

Bobby McFerrin

An advertising brochure was on the kitchen table and Bernie read the cover, "Are you Worried About Losing Your Memory?"

"Naw," he joked, "not me, I don't have a memory!"

He got a big kiss and a hug for that!

Blow-Up At The Mall

Jace took Bernie on the bus to the mall, and I only know what he told me.

Things were going along really well when Bernie got very upset. It may have been all the hustle and bustle, people all stirring and moving about, strange faces and lots of noise but when he suddenly couldn't find me, he kept asking, "Where's Betty Lee? Where's my wife?" He raised his voice, yelling, "Where's my wife?" Poor Jace, he was really frightened and tried to phone me, but I must have been outside, I didn't hear the ring.

He was afraid to take Bernie back on the bus, so he got him into a taxi. Bernie just kept yelling and kicking the back of the driver's seat. The driver must have thought Bernie was crazy and told Jace he wouldn't take them any further, but Jace persisted and he finally brought them home.

Well, that sure didn't work out and there were no more buses and no more visits to the mall without me. I think large, strange crowds frighten him when I 'm not there.

I also worried what people would think about Bernie. On occasion he'd talk to a driver in the car next to us at a signal, and sometimes start to open his door to get out and continue the conversation. So I had to keep the doors locked. Also, he always talked to children and pets, and I was concerned that some parent might think he was up to no good, or someone, somehow might take something the wrong way and lash out at him.

One day we got caught up in a restaurant doorway and a young punk in front turned and snarled at me that I had 'dissed' him. I pulled Bernie with me as I moved away. I was afraid he might have said or done the wrong thing, he didn't normally take lightly to a challenge from thugs. I tried to watch out for him when we were in public--just one more thing to be concerned about.

Return to Royale Park

I couldn't think of anyplace better to bring Bernie after his improvements than back to Royale Park. I wanted to see how the staff would react. I was not disappointed.

Everyone was astonished; many of them had tears in their eyes. After all, they lose most of their patients, so to see one get better had to be an emotional high. More than one mentioned that they had never noticed what beautiful eyes Bernie had. That didn't surprise me, Alzheimer's patients rarely make eye contact and often have their eyes downcast.

Bernie was completely overcome by the experience. He had no idea why everyone was so kind to him, shaking his hand, touching his arm, caring so much. He became very emotional, his face turned red and I could see tears forming. He didn't cry, but his face got all twisted up--the attention was too much.

Apparently, he didn't remember any of the people or the facility and yet, as I walked to the front door ahead of him, he tarried behind in the lobby as if he was going to stay. When I stepped back to collect him--Scottie, his old girlfriend, was already leading him away.

Giving Us A Bad Time

Although Bernie continued to improve rapidly in some areas, in others, he hadn't budged an inch. He still got very angry when Jace tried to change his clothes. He still pulled his clothes on if we were trying to take them off, or took them off while we were trying to put them on. It was especially true in the morning when Jace wanted to take off his pajamas. He really pulled to keep them on and got red-in-the-face angry, making a sometime fist--that seems to be typical of Alzheimer's--some sort of common reflex. Thankfully, he wasn't doing it as often and I could take the fist, give it a little kiss and that made it relax. It was frightening because someone who didn't know his condition could misread that fist--like a stranger at the mall or someone jostled in a doorway.

I'd try to divert Bernie's attention, to get his hands busy with something else so that he'd let go of his clothes. I'd tell him how handsome he was, how much I loved him, gave him lots of kisses, but it was a real struggle. Because he had a lot of trouble figuring out how to sit down, it sometimes took both Jace and me to get him seated, and that, too, could upset him.

A care agency once told me that caring for an Alzheimer's patient is worse than for any other condition. It is the hardest, the quickest to cause burnout, it's completely exhausting, demanding and relentless. Another doctor told me that many professional caregivers for at-home Alzheimer's patients now refuse to work if they're the only one on duty. She said it takes two people full time to care for one patient 24/7--as if I needed to be told any of that!

So I tried to see that Jace didn't get overwhelmed. I told him to come to me immediately, no matter what I was doing, if he had a problem. Together, we were doing the best we could.

My Job

Mostly Jace took care of Bernie and did it very well. I was pleased and relieved about that. My job though, as I saw it, was to be with Bernie. I absolutely believed that being at home was best for him, except for not having the social stimulation he'd had at Royale. I'd sit with him a lot on the couch, just holding and kissing his hand, or with my head on his shoulder to keep reinforcing positive feelings in him, to encourage, to spoil, to love. I let him see me all the time. I knew he was frightened before and still after the surgery, and I was frightened, too. He didn't ask, but I told him he'd been sick, that he'd had an operation and was getting better.

He had to feel great uncertainty about himself, knowing he couldn't really do anything, could barely make a coherent sentence--he had to feel insecure. So I thought I had to make him feel worthwhile--which he was to me anyway--tell him how important he was to a lot of people and show him he was truly loved. He had to come to have faith that I would always be there for him, keeping him safe and secure. It was a new role for both of us--but if wasn't me, then who?

When he'd come looking for me, I'd stop whatever I was doing to be with him. I talked to him, teased him, told him again how handsome he was, and he liked to hear all of that. Sometimes I'd talk about old times, the children, the house. He was beginning to ask a lot more for Matt, wanted to talk to him, see him. I thought he was used to the time they'd spent together in the garage, Matt's shop, or at the racetrack. When I talked about France, Debby and her family, he'd forget our ever having been there even when I showed him photos of us with them in her house. But he liked to pet 'Sophie' called her to him, talked to her.

At the same time, if Jace was in another room and Bernie heard a sound, he'd ask if someone was in the house, he kept forgetting about Jace's being there, and he couldn't remember Jace's name. But he always recognized him when he saw him, and he showed great affection and appreciation to him for the way he cared for him. They developed a male bond, and that was good for both.

I'd always been very comfortable being with Bernie and those moments with him were more precious to me than ever. But I needed my 'alone' time as well, and with Jace, I could take it.

Adult Day Care

As the days went on and more of his awareness returned he was restless and bored, so I took him to an adult day care program for others like him. There were about fifteen people, all with some form of dementia. While Bernie would have been too far gone and unable to participate only a few months before, he was now right in the thick of it.

Interacting with other people, especially the man to man stuff stimulated him. His speech seemed less garbled, he was friendly, well liked, flirted with the ladies, and had a sly smile when I teased him about it--the 'ole' dog. And while he did some things well, he was unable to follow enough to play Bingo.

Sometimes he'd be agitated there and kept asking, "Where's my wife?" Other times he'd pace and, when these things happened, I let them give him half a Xanax. They said he calmed down in 15 to 20 minutes. Sometimes I did the same at home. I really appreciated having adult day care and their ever-patient staff. It made a positive difference in him and in my opportunity to have free time.

However, I never told him he was going to day care, instead I'd say 'they called and need you at work.' Briefly I'd tell him what he'd be doing and name a few of the people. He began to feel important and useful. Sometimes we'd go through a dialogue about work--he'd say with mock annoyance, 'work, work, work, but it has to be done.' He'd display a little phony resignation when the van pulled up but gave the driver a friendly hello, and off he went with a smile of anticipation. "They're waiting for me," he'd explain.

A Well Deserved Gift

I've heard any number of people wish for just one more day, one more hour to be with a loved one they have lost, or in a situation like Bernie's, to communicate, to understand, to respond once again.

So this wish came true for me, and I didn't intend to waste it. No matter what else happened, I had been given this time to say all the things I ever wanted to say, give all the hugs and kisses I needed to give, share all the laughter. Over and over I'd tell him how much I appreciated all he did for me and the children, how proud I was of the part he played in the space program, how much I loved him, always loved him, always would--and he just glowed.

I could also be upset, however, by his annoying personality traits that were returning, telling me how to drive, taking over, interrupting. I sometimes wished I could have been able to pick and choose the qualities I wanted to see return and leave the others behind, but then he wouldn't be my Bernie, would he? And *zhoh*, I intended to appreciate all of it! In no small way, I loved Bernie more than ever. Maybe it was because he was so vulnerable, and I could dote on him endlessly. Anyway, God knows he'd been through enough hell and damnation for too many years, he deserved this gift--and so did I!

◆TWENTY-SIX◆

May 1999

The Video

As Bernie regained his strength, and I noticed all the subtle changes, I thought about the video I'd made before surgery and devised a video test to show his current progress. I remembered how he'd been unable to select something out of a group, so I put some random items on the kitchen table and asked him to hand a specific one to me. He was unable to do it. A month later, I tried again. This time he was a little better, but not much. When I filmed the third month after surgery, he was substantially better. By the fourth month, he was downright perfect and Jace even put him on a bicycle. That's when I looked at the whole video for the first time.

Until I saw the tape, I didn't realize the profound sadness and despair Bernie had shown at Royale. I could watch the beginning of the video only because I knew he was now so much better. Otherwise, I'd have thrown it away, it was breaking my heart. Most people were unable to watch it at all, leaving the room in tears or asking me to turn it off. As each month of the selection game came on screen, I began to realize what a remarkable thing had been recorded. In four months he'd gone from barely having a life to riding a bicycle and laughing about it.

I immediately made a copy and sent it to Dr. Goldsmith, who was obviously very pleased. The truth is, the doctor really didn't know Bernie. The man in the video was a complete stranger to him, nothing at all like the wraith he'd first seen in Royale Park. It's important for the reader to realize that Bernie still had Alzheimer's, always would, it's just that his life was so vastly improved. An indication of how he still had the disease was when I played the tape for him. He had no memory of being in his room at Royale. The courtyard was visible in the video, but he didn't recognize that either. He never understood that he ever left home for any reason.

When he watched the video and heard my voice asking him to do something on the tape, he'd get up from his chair and go do what I asked him to do on camera. He answered my voice on the video without understanding that I was sitting next to him at the same time. It was pretty funny, actually quite charming, if it wasn't so sad. He did that a lot, confused what was happening on the TV with reality, even when it was his own image on the screen.

Harry was sending the video to his medical colleagues and I'd begun sending it to the media. I told Bernie that the video had been seen by people all over the country, even abroad. Remembering what the German doctor thought, I said that he may be famous one day, even on TV.

"Really?"

"Really."

"Wow," he smiled. "I must be pretty important."

Well, anyway, I thought, you are to me.

July 1999

Six Months After Surgery

Two Thumbs Up

Deb arrived from France with Guillaume and Justin for a short summer visit. I was looking forward to their seeing Bernie, noting the contrast between this year and last. Of course, they'd seen the video, knew he was more aware and looking better.

While they were here, she told me that she asked the boys what they thought of the change in Big Daddy and they gave him 'two thumbs up.' You can't get a better review than that!

That having been said, I decided to increase my attempts at going public--I really thought it was important. So far I hadn't had any response to the videos I'd sent out. Harry seemed to think I was wasting my time, he'd been trying to get interest in the omentum going for years.

Black And Blank

As Bernie regained more awareness, I thought it frightened him when he realized something was happening. The most likely time he'd talk about it was when we were in bed.

"I can't *do* anything," he'd tell me. And he was right. Sometimes he couldn't even put a plate on the table. "I can't take care of you anymore." He was devastated.

"I know," I told him. I didn't argue with the things he believed, much less the things that were real. "But you've taken care of me and the kids for fifty years, and you did a wonderful job, now it's my turn to take care of you, and that's what I'm doing, and that's what I want to do."

"But I'm so frightened."

"I know, but I'm here, I'll always be here, and 'Sophie' is here, and Debby and the boys, and Matt and Zeli. We're all OK, and nothing bad is going to happen, I promise."

I know I'd said those things before--not only to him--I remember saying them to the children when they were little and something bad happened in their lives. "Don't worry, I'll always be here." One never knows, of course, but it's what you have to say to bring comfort to someone in fear, even though you know it might not happen that way. But you play the odds in life, after all they're in your favor.

"I'm frightened," he'd tell me. "I don't know who I am, I have no memory."

"Don't you know your name?"

"Yes, I'm Bernhardt."

"Yes, you're Bernhardt. Do you know who I am?"

"Of course, you're Betty Lee, my wife."

"And don't you remember when we went to school together?"

"No, I don't remember Dorsey (our high school)." That brought a little self-conscious laugh as he realized what he'd said about our high school. "I told you I didn't remember Dorsey, but that's what I remembered!"

I can't explain how he remembered something he said he didn't remember. Maybe he just got his words all twisted, but he remembered. When a story about landing on the moon was on TV, I asked if he remembered that he'd made a transformer for it, and he remembered that right away. Sometimes he'd remember something and sometimes not. It began to make me think that he acted like people I'd seen on TV who have amnesia. His memory was like a checkerboard, but instead of black and red, it's black and blank.

"What happened to me?" I'd tell him he had a problem with his memory but he was getting better all the time, that we took him to Germany and had surgery to help him get better. I told him this many, many times, but it was always fresh news and a wonderment to him.

It had to be terrifying. I couldn't even begin to image what it's like to have no memory of what has just happened, to have only scattered memories of the past, and no idea what will happen in the next minute, to not know who you are. It isn't only that you're living in the mini-moment, it's being lost in a mental outer space, you don't know which way the earth is, where to find the moon. You can't contact Houston if you have a problem, there are no directions, it's all just empty--empty and terrifying.

Surgery In The States

No one was going to do anything about getting the surgery done in the States. If no one would stick their necks out to do it on behalf of Harry, why would they do it for me? I knew any number of doctors who had seen Bernie's tape and who were not opposed to the procedure, so I called one to talk about my hopes of having the surgery done here, going abroad was too hard on the patients. He stunned me by saying that even if it were possible, it would take at least three or four years! I couldn't believe it, I just couldn't believe it! Bernie had shown enough progress that it was worth pursuing and I didn't understand why we couldn't do it next week! In three or four years thousands of people will die. Why can't we help some of them now?

He began to explain by introducing me into the world of protocols, institutional review boards (IRB), conflicts, personalities, procedures, legalities, delays, and more. Of course he was right, but at the time I didn't know what he was talking about. I hung up feeling somber, unsettled and annoyed. There didn't seem to be much opportunity there, not the way I wanted it anyway.

August 1999

Growing Awareness

Bernie was easier for me to care for. Jace no longer lived with us and only worked during the day. But Bernie's sometime anger frightened and upset him, so I rarely left them alone. I'm sure part of it was having another man in the house. Bernie's face could turn deep red, he'd threaten with his fist and shake with rage, but it was different than before the surgery, I could always talk him down. He'd apologize, saying he'd never hurt me, Jace or anyone else. I took that all as progress, that his awareness of his behavior was improving

His anger surfaced when he was asked to do something that confused him, it wasn't just random. If I wanted him to take off his shirt, he'd unbutton, then rebutton it, so I'd try to guide him, and that sort of thing, his needing help with his clothes, could easily anger him. Yet, if I helped him to remove his shirt in a doctor's office, he never got angry. With returning awareness, he was making conscious decisions because sometimes I could see that a lot of it was bravado.

In many ways he was quite helpless and that resulted in his being treated like a child, which he no doubt resented. Jace and I tried to give him his dignity and control, but it wasn't always possible. You can only accommodate someone with dementia so much, and you'll just have to trust me on that.

One afternoon, returning from a walk with Jace and 'Sophie,' he came in the backdoor all distressed, telling me he didn't know why he'd behaved in such a terrible way. Jace told me that Bernie had seen a car like mine and waved. When the driver didn't stop or wave back, he just began to seethe. Maybe he thought I was ignoring him, but he realized his actions were foolish and he felt chagrined. Then he apologized to Jace, saying that he was sorry and offering his hand to shake.

I knew that I was the one tangible touch he had with his reality. It had to be a horror for him when I was not around, but it was hard on me, too. So, since he'd been behaving better, I went out for a couple of hours. It didn't work. When I got home, Jace said Bernie was really angry, had grabbed his wrists and pushed things around on the table, but he never really hurt him. I didn't know if that was escalation or not, only time would tell. For the rest of the day, Bernie was upset. He didn't want Jace in the house, he didn't like *any* men in the house.

Sometimes I'd ask Jace to go walk around the block so Bernie couldn't see him for a while--but I didn't like to do that. Finally, I told Bernie that Jace had to be here to help me and he'd just have to learn to live with it. All I did was make it worse. It was a big mistake to challenge him, and I knew it, but that's what I did anyway.

I've done so many stupid, wrong things in life--I'm not about to list them--but this was just one more dumb--should have known better--big boo-boo.

More Paranoia

It is not unusual for Alzheimer's patients to be paranoid and Bernie still had mini-bouts of that. One evening he determined that something was terribly wrong and it had to be taken care of immediately. It turned out to be a chest of drawers in Debby's room that had to be moved. I told him we'd take care of it first thing in the morning, but he insisted it had to be done *now*. I was in no mood to start moving furniture around. There were some items on top, so I picked them up and said, "You're right, we'll start with these right now. Let's put them in the kitchen." I put everything on the kitchen counter and started talking about something else. Within minutes Bernie had forgotten what terrible dangers lurked in the bureau.

I never knew what his fertile imagination would conjure up next, and each incident required a different approach. You can't talk an Alzheimer's patient out of what he actually knows to be real, so you always agree and then figure out something that will satisfy the moment, knowing that he'll forget soon enough. If I had argued that there was nothing dangerous about the chest of drawers, he'd have insisted that there was, he'd get angry, the whole thing would be blown out of proportion and there'd be another scene. It was just easier to lie outright, to fabricate whatever scenario worked.

Another evening he came to me all shaking and terrified, saying that 'they' were going to kill him. Of course, he couldn't tell me who, when or why, but I went into the den where he'd been sitting and there was a scary movie on TV. I turned it off, then got into bed with him, put a classical concert on TV and laid there holding his hand. He soon fell asleep. I tried to be alert to what might cause these things to begin with, I didn't think it all just came out of nowhere.

August 1999

Matt & Zeli Have A Party

Matt and Zeli were so happy together, so crazy about each other, it was a joy to see. Of course, they'd only been married eight months. They loved to entertain, especially a backyard bar-b-que with way too much food.

So that's what they did, their first big event since they married, and most of the guests, about 30 or so, had been at their wedding where they'd last seen Bernie and me. The whole afternoon was a battery of stunned expressions, mouths agape, jaws dropping open, they couldn't believe it, they simply could not believe that Bernie was the same man they'd pitied at the wedding.

Over and over again, one by one, in twos and threes, they came up to us, often with moist eyes, marveling at Matt's Dad, so different from the wretched man they'd seen only months before, so healthy, so vital, so aware. And Bernie loved it, every minute.

So here was an impartial jury if ever there was one. Many guests were from childhood, boys I had watched grow up with Matt, friends from college, racing buddies, Zeli's friends, all knew him in one way or another, some for a lifetime, others just recently, but to a man--and to a woman--they were happy and amazed. It validated everything I'd been through, and as Bernie himself had said to me, "Ya done good."

I'd been thinking that Bernie went from advanced Alzheimer's back to moderate Alzheimer's, and just days ago, Matt told me that he thought his Dad was at about the same spot he was two years ago, well before we placed him in Royale Park. Since I'd been thinking the same thing, I felt it must be a fairly accurate assessment.

Moving On

Thankfully, Bernie never did wander. In fact, after surgery it was months before he even went into the backyard alone. Now he went in the front yard, but never left the immediate area of our house. He could start to do that, I hoped not, but for the moment I thought he was afraid.

He'd also always fed himself and still did, although on occasion he needed a little help to get started or complete a meal, especially breakfast, but seldom in a restaurant--or if it was something sweet--he'd scrape the platter clean. Every month or so he appeared to lose weight and I'd bulk him up again with his adult supplement. I believed that was still the Alzheimer's, they do lose weight. He moved slow much of the time, nurtured that humongous sweet tooth, and folded paper napkins into his pockets, all odd symptoms of Alzheimer's. Otherwise, when I took him for a check-up to his primary physician, all tests showed he was physically fine

Still, I knew that this progressive degenerating disease would always be there--but not like it would have been without the surgery--because there'd just been so much incredible improvement. If I didn't have Jace to help I couldn't do it alone anymore, I was aging and burning out. But if things continued to improve, in a few months or so I didn't think I'd need someone all day, maybe a few hours in the morning, and then he could go to adult day care most afternoons.

Knocking On Media Doors

With a little more free time now, I'd begun calling newspapers, the Health Section of the Los Angeles Times to begin with, then every other section I thought would have an interest. Boy, was I naïve. I thought surely they'd want to do a story--'Local Man Reverses Alzheimer's Symptoms'--but they were polite, said they'd get back to me--of course, they didn't. Neither did other newspapers, magazines, AARP, senior this and senior that, not a peep from any TV talk show, nothing, no interest whatsoever. I followed up with phone calls, personal letters, more videos, but I couldn't get anywhere--just as Harry said it would be. I avoided radio talk shows though. I knew that if I just opened my mouth on the air, the host could immediately tear me down and then all the negativity would be out there--and the media loves the negative.

I was tempted to buy a newspaper ad, but that would look like Harry was trolling for patients, and nothing was further from the truth. Harry kept telling me not to bother, he'd been down this road too many times, I wouldn't be able to do it. Nonetheless, I promised him that I'd find a backdoor. I'd done years of publicity for volunteer organizations--*I knew how to do this!* Except, I wasn't getting anywhere! I didn't understand how anyone--everyone--could ignore such an important issue.

•TWENTY-SEVEN•

September 3, 1999

"On A Slow Boat To China"

Frank Loesser, 1948

That's what Bernie always told me fifty years ago when we were dating as teen-agers, "I'd like to get you on a slow boat to China." He'd sing it to me, hum it in my ear on those few occasions if it played when we danced, whisper it, and I would have been happy enough to sail with him. Of course, it never came to pass, and that's just as well, I think we'd have both been seasick--not terribly romantic. Instead we had reasonably smooth sailing in our little symbolic marital canoe on the sea of life until we were capsized by Alzheimer's. Only last year, on our 48th wedding anniversary I was visiting him in the 'Cuckoo's Nest.' We'd been scuttled and I'd told everyone that there weren't going to be any more anniversary celebrations for us, never again--and now, this stunning turnaround!!! Who woulda thunk it?

So this year, Matt and Zeli took us out for an elegant anniversary brunch, except that the restaurant I'd chosen wasn't serving brunch that day so we ended up at our usual coffee shop. And you know what? It was grand, it was just downright grand!

And it gave me an idea that I knew was going to work, oh, you can bet it was going to work!

November 1999

"It's Kinda Fun To Do The Impossible."

Walt Disney

Although they routinely run this type of story, the Los Angeles Times couldn't have cared less about Bernie and the surgery. A publisher of hospital newsletters told me that it would never be accepted by anyone because it had not been scientifically proven, it was all anecdotal. Everyone was afraid of lawsuits, going against the establishment, jeopardizing their careers, yada, yada, yada.

A friend in medicine warned, "Be careful, Betty, the medical establishment is a formidable foe."

"My husband has Alzheimer's," I countered, "what can they do to me?"

With a self-imposed mission to complete, I didn't care about all this silliness, and dismissed it upon hearing. Besides I had found the media's backdoor, so with a copy of a snapshot taken of Bernie and me at Matt and Zeli's party, I sent this release to the one place I knew there'd be no editorial rejection--the Society Section of the Los Angeles Times.

"Bernie and Betty Weiss of Westchester, childhood sweethearts from grade school through graduation from Dorsey High School, celebrated their 49th wedding anniversary on Sept. 3 with special joy.

Last year, Bernie was confined to an institution, suffering with advanced Alzheimer's disease. Today, after successful surgery in Germany, the majority of his symptoms have reversed themselves. He lives again at home, and enjoys their children, Debby, Jean-François, Matt and Zeli, and grandchildren Guillaume and Justin.

Bernie founded the Zenith Transformer Co., designing and manufacturing transformers for all the early space shots. One unit still remains on the moon. Betty, a lifelong volunteer, ran the training program at LAX's Traveler's Aid Society for 13 years."

They printed it, and just like that I was in and never looked back.

I left a lot of clues to find us--that we lived in the Westchester section of Los Angeles, our school and work. People called others they knew from Dorsey and Traveler's Aid to ask about us--if this was really legit. I got cards from classmates, and Bernie's former employees. Some readers called the Times directly to contact me. You'd be surprised who looks at the society pages.

As the calls came in, I knew the callers had rehearsed what they were going to say, after all, who calls a stranger to wish them well on their 49th wedding anniversary?

"Oh, Mrs. Weiss," they'd begin, "I just wanted to tell you how wonderful I think it is to see a couple married so long in this day and age." (Long pause.) "But you know, there was something else I just happened to notice in the article---." Then I'd hear their poignant stories. Some called to tell me about their loved ones who had already died, but they were so glad to hear there may be something out there to help others.

They told friends and family in other states about it, including doctors who also called me.

I listened to everyone, sent them copies of my research papers and videotapes, gave them Dr. Goldsmith's phone number, and told our story over and over. At about 30 calls, I stopped counting and changed my answering machine message, asking callers to please leave a phone number and I'd get back to them. I couldn't keep up the non-stop talking. Maybe editors and the medical establishment weren't interested, but look at the calls I got from a comment buried in an article appearing, of all places, in the society pages.

But there were unforeseen problem. I had no idea at the time that in Germany, Dr. Goldsmith's colleague had left Bathildis to practice at another hospital, and because he had so much confidence in this one doctor, his medical skills and English speaking abilities, he didn't feel comfortable in Bad Pyrmont operating without him, so he was going to make other arrangements. I was hoping that would mean the States, avoiding airplanes.

Now that people knew about it, I felt awful because there was no place for them to go. In a couple of weeks, the calls trickled away. I had no clue about what to do next. And, besides, for the moment I had other problems to deal with.

Escalating

Bernie got more and more paranoid about Jace and 'them.' One morning he kicked at him, didn't really hurt him, but it was a bad thing to do. He just didn't like 'them' in the house and it was all being taken out on Jace. I don't want to give the impression that Bernie was still violent or as paranoid as he was before surgery, he wasn't, not by a long shot, he was not like that at all. After the surgery, he never kicked anyone, never hit anyone, never even threatened anyone else--he was just fixated on Jace.

Finally, one morning I came running to the kitchen, hearing screams from Bernie. "I've got one, I've got one!" He was holding Jace by the arm and threatening to cut off his head with a frying pan. Bernie never hurt him in any way, and although Jace could have easily decked him, he understood what was happening and didn't even try. Still he left that day and I didn't blame him.

The paranoia, seeing himself in a distant mirror, hearing normal household sounds--to Bernie, it was all 'them' in the house. I just hoped it would lessen as time went on. I was reluctant to try any drugs because they always made him worse and things just weren't that bad. I always believed that we'd have had less of a problem if he'd had the surgery sooner, before the paranoia got such a tight grip on him.

Thanksgiving

With Thanksgiving looming, I thought I'd have a lot to be grateful for, that Bernie was so much better, and doing so remarkably well, although all along he'd have brief set-backs. Then I'd think he was reverting and that it was all for naught, but he always came around after a few minutes, or at the most, a few hours.

Ten months after surgery, he had another setback, and this time he went backwards so fast it was like he stepped off a cliff. By the second day, I was really worried. He'd begun to stoop, his eyes became dull and the lids were drooping. He was agitated and bristling, lost bowel control, and was particularly upset when a painter, another man, was in the house. Everything just slowed down, he was almost back to where he was when I had to place him. I was so worried, so worried. I called the doctor monitoring his meds and he put him on Aricept. Then I watched him closer than ever--would he improve? Oh, please, please, oh, please let him improve.

All along I kept thinking that we at least had these ten months--and they were good months. He'd been to some parties, we ate out, went to the movies, did all the ordinary things that people do. Besides gaining almost all bowel control, he had a normal sleep pattern, he didn't fall--even when balancing on one leg to put on his pants--he was walking tall, eyes were alert--he was participating in life--things had been going so well, and now this. Suppose he kept going downhill?

My mind bounced around between thinking about his having to be placed again or his getting better. Maybe I could get full time help in the house again and not place him. I couldn't rehire Jace, of course, although that would have been my preference, but it couldn't be a man. The hours were crawling by and then--just as quickly--it all turned around and within four days, he was back to his improved self--almost. Physically he was alert again, improving in his behavior skills, but he'd lost some of his long-term memory. I don't understand how he could improve in one area and lose ground in another, but overall, he was still improving, so I couldn't complain. If it has to be, I prefer it this way, that his behavior improves, I can live with some memory loss.

Was it just a prolonged and deeper setback than the others, or did the Aricept catch it just in time? Maybe he had a mini-stroke or something else happened, I didn't know how we'd ever know.

December 1999

"Something Is Rotten In The State Of Denmark"

'Marcellus'
"Hamlet"

All this time, the tape I'd made was being sent to people who should have embraced it, but instead didn't even look at it, or if they did it was challenged. Debby showed it to doctors in France. Mostly they dismissed it with contempt. One said it couldn't be true because he didn't see any surgical scars on Bernie. I was astonished to learn that people thought it had to leave grotesque scars--how or why I couldn't imagine. At a family support group, the doctor there had the nerve to tell Debby, in front of other suffering families, that it was impossible.

An eminent doctor on the faculty of a southern university called me on the phone a couple of times and sent me a copy of a letter he'd written to the Vice President for Medicine and Science for the Alzheimer's Association.

He mentioned Bernie and the other Alzheimer's patients having had the surgery, arguing that '*the clinical observations...requires the particular and immediate attention of your organization...even this limited series of the above patients, presents evidence that as researchers and clinicians we have to clinically look at AD as a disease of microcirculation...while I agree that the clinical problem of AD is not solely based on a blood flow problem...this approach can more rapidly provide us with a clinical route to improving mentation and reversing AD pathology.*'

'*I know that in this day and age that another "Semmelweiss"* (Hungarian obstetrician, 1818-65, ridiculed and rejected for advocating that doctors wash their hands between patients.) *debacle is considered by our colleagues in medicine and the public to be impossible.*

However...the press (i.e; Newsweek, TV, the L.A. Times, etc.) ignore requests for review and presentation because of clinical advisors who with prejudice shrug off his (Goldsmith's) work as "anecdotal, not possessed of adequate preclinical study, etc." without fair review...I am sorry to say that there is a microcirculatory prejudice...alive and well among our Neuroscience colleagues.'

So it wasn't just my feelings of unease that something else was going on--this was a missive from someone on the inside that verified there was something--use your own description--a conspiracy, a vendetta, an ignorance, an arrogance, a laziness, a jealousy, financial greed--a widespread something unspoken that did not have the patient's well being at heart.

I called the medical reporter who wrote the article I'd first read and told her how well Bernie was doing. I was sure that her magazine would be interested in a follow-up, since it was in their publication that the story first broke, they could do a little well-deserved crowing. I sent her a write-up of all his improvements, she got together with her agent who agreed it was a shoo-in--and it was turned down flat! I was beginning to understand the total silence. Apparently any doctor in an advisory capacity for the media is pre-programmed to shut the door on omentum transposition and Dr. Goldsmith. Again, no one was interested in Bernie and finding out how his experience might help others.

The history of Dr. Semmelweiss and doctors washing their hands is supposed to be taught to all medical students so that they will always keep an open mind to new theories as they come along--to possibly save lives. That lesson doesn't seem to be getting through--minds are as closed as ever. Further, if it really is being taught, it's worse than just shuttered minds, it's being ignored in practice as well--since it is well documented that a substantial number of modern doctors, even knowing the risks, still don't wash their own hands--it seems to be too much of a bother.

In the German hospital, every room had a small dispenser on the wall. It contained a gel-like antiseptic that dried immediately. Doctors automatically used it as they left a patient before going on to the next one. Some facilities may be using it here, although I haven't yet seen it, but it certainly should be universally required. (http://www.institute-shot.com/hand_washing_by_health_care_providers.htm)

I received calls from other doctors who had chosen not to go public--and who could blame them? Why should they subject themselves to the same batterings that Dr. Goldsmith has endured?

A prominent doctor from another world famous university called. We talked for nearly an hour, he asked me question after question. How did I find out about this? What made me think it would work? He really made me delve into my memory--to relive the research, my beliefs, my emotions. Finally he said, "Well, your reasoning was sound." That impressed me no end, because anyone in the field would recognize his name if I felt free to mention it, and I asked, "If that's the case, why does the medical profession reject it?" "Because," he answered, "we doctors don't like it when someone comes out of left field and tells us something we should have seen for ourselves years ago." Ah, now there was an honest man!

Traci

With Jace gone, I really didn't need anyone to help with Bernie. But it was nearly seven years since he was first diagnosed with short-term memory loss, and I felt like I was out of breath, as if I'd been running all this time for dear life. I was fortunate to have the resources to hire help and so I did. I know too many other caregivers don't have those options--and they need it, not just for Alzheimer's, but for dozens of other long-term medical conditions. It's too hard if you're all alone getting older and your loved one is only going to worsen.

Traci was from Belize, and arrived like a Christmas gift for me. She came in at 7:00 a.m., prepared our breakfast, tidied the kitchen, saw that Bernie was dressed and groomed--that takes 20 minutes or so--showers a little longer. Then she did the laundry, went food shopping, prepared dinner, and was on her way home in three or four hours, often dropping him off at day care. I don't know why it took me the better part of a century to figure out that I could have someone come in to shop and cook. What a joy--and I deserved *that*, too.

I know how hard it would have been for me if I didn't have help, and I know there are those who have no help and those who refuse to get any help--even when it's available, affordable and offered. I think it's even harder when you're the caregiver for a parent, trying to raise children, maybe working, and finding time for your spouse. Since it was only Bernie and me, I wasn't being pulled in all directions, but I still had a lot to do.

I was alone with him only very little in the mornings, but I was always with him after day care until he went to bed. I still had the responsibility of the house and yard, 'Sophie,' maintaining the car, paying the bills, marketing because Traci only did some of the food shopping, and only Bernie's laundry. I had endless errands, the bank, the cleaners, getting us both to doctor appointments and 'Sophie' to the vet, seeing that Bernie got his hair cut, and all the myriad things that everyone else has to do--and sometimes I just liked to *do nothing*--and when I had the chance, that's what I did--because anyone who is a home-bound caregiver for an Alzheimer's loved one must be able to labor like Hercules, have the patience of Job, the wisdom of Solomon, the physical strength of Samson, the endurance of a Marathoner, the sensitivity of a butterfly, the hide of a rhino, take the punishment of an anvil, be gentle as a soap bubble, remain forever vigilant, constantly alert, never sleep, dismiss one's own needs, eliminate everything and everyone else, and have faith that the sun will shine again. Other than that, there's not much to it.

Well, that's the way it used to be before surgery, now I was often strolling down easy street.

Traci and Bernie were very comfortable together, and he was no longer paranoid--didn't see 'them' anymore. I thought a lot if it had to do with having a woman in the house and not another man--or maybe, hopefully, there was just less paranoia as a result of the surgery. All in all, and in spite of my frequent worries, Bernie was just so much better living at home, needing supervision--that's true, but doing really well. It has to take time for new blood vessels to form, to fight the valiant fight, and Alzheimer's is an evil, vile adversary--one must give the devil his due.

A Disney Adventure

We were going for a walk, the three of us--Bernie, 'Sophie' and me. We were out the backdoor, all ready,

Bernie in race hat and jacket was holding 'Sophie' who was sporting her new blue leash. I went back inside to get a sun hat.

"Wait right here, don't go away." I admonished them on the driveway. "Stay!"

I don't think I was inside for more than a few moments, but they were gone when I came back out. I wasn't terribly concerned. I knew they were just taking their usual route around the block, so I got in the car to go after them.

Except I didn't see them! I knew that both Jace and Traci had taken them on long walks all around the neighborhood, even as far as the park, so 'Sophie' may not be staying on the block any more. I made wider and wider circles, looking down all the streets, asking the mailman, gardeners, others out walking, "Have you seen a man and a big brown dog?"

No one had seen them. I went by the shopping center, but didn't see them. Maybe they went into a store, someone's house, they could have been anyplace. I drove back past the house, but they hadn't returned. I could have asked the neighbors to help search or call Matt, but by the time he got here, they could be in another county. I drove further and further away making bigger and bigger circles, asking, looking, checking the park, but there was no sign of them. Bernie had his Medic Alert bracelet, so if someone found him they'd have a number to call, but I was worried anyway. I thought I could rely on 'Sophie' to bring them back, and she had her ID tag, but suppose they got separated?

After a half-hour or more of a fruitless effort, I decided to call the police--I couldn't do this alone. Mentally, I was describing them, what Bernie was wearing, and 'Sophie's blue leash--what to tell the police.

God, how could I lose them!

But when I drove up the driveway to make the phone call, there they were at the backdoor. I hugged them both and Bernie's torso was warm, his face shiny. 'Sophie' dragged herself inside, slurped at her water dish and immediately flopped down. Oh, they'd been someplace, that was for sure, they were both so hot and tired. They'd had an adventure.

"Where've you been?"

"I don't know," Bernie answered.

And 'Sophie' wasn't talking.

◆TWENTY-EIGHT◆

January 2000

"In The Future Everyone Will Be Famous For Fifteen Minutes"

Andy Warhol

"All Right, Mr. DeMille, I'm Ready For My Close-Up"

Norma Desmond
"Sunset Boulevard," 1950

One last person called me about our 'anniversary' article, Drew Griffin, a television reporter in Los Angeles for CBS, (He currently reports for CNN.) He did "Special Assignment" segments on Sunday nights, just before "60 Minutes." His father-in-law had advanced Alzheimer's disease. He'd never heard of the surgery and, like the others, had a lot of questions. I answered everything he asked and as I'd been doing for everyone else, sent him articles and the tape, expecting nothing would come of it once again. He never mentioned doing an interview, he seemed like just one more interested party with an afflicted family member. I wasn't sure of his motivation and didn't ask about an interview. Would CBS nix it, anyway? But, when he wanted Harry's phone number, I gave it to him.

A few days later, Harry was telling me that a reporter from Los Angeles wanted to do an interview, but he didn't want to do it because he'd had so much bad publicity in the past and his detractors would take out after him again. This made me stop and think, too. While I wanted to do it, and didn't mind any accolades, I didn't want to appear as if I were Harry's shill, and more than that, I didn't want to embarrass Bernie--because Alzheimer's is an embarrassing disease. But, of course, this is what I'd been working for, going to the public while always knowing that eventually I'd have to put Bernie on display--and I really had these mixed feelings.

I remember how hard it was to talk about Bernie and Alzheimer's for so many years, but once I crossed the threshold and went up front with it, I didn't feel such reluctant embarrassment--it was rather liberating, to be honest. Like with every mental illness, many families still keep Alzheimer's a secret, protecting and hiding the victim as much as possible--there's all that understandable denial. Now we'd really be exposed to the world, like Reagan's family, although obviously there wouldn't be all the fanfare. It'd be different, but they could still make us look bad--it'd be easy enough to do.

Several phone calls now ensued among Drew, Harry and me. I asked Matt and Debby if they thought Dad would be OK with it if he had full awareness, and they said yes. I thought so, too, but I told Harry it was up to him. I knew that this was the only chance we'd have to make it public--it was Drew or nothing--probably ever. I certainly didn't have any more tricks in my little bag. But if I didn't continue to push for it, let the public see Bernie, then who would? We had to do the interview if anything was to be accomplished.

President Reagan

As important as it was for Reagan to go public, I didn't feel the true Alzheimer's story was getting out. He'd be all neatly dressed, walking in a nearby park, waving to other strollers, stopping to have his picture taken, looking so hale and hearty--and it was all so misleading. Not that I was blaming anyone. As I said, families do everything possible to shield their loved ones, to keep them looking good and as normal as possible. The problem with Reagan was that the public saw him that way and said, "So that's Alzheimer's, how bad can it be?"

Certainly I am not suggesting that the public be allowed to see Reagan doing all I've written about Bernie--the things every caregiver knows both men said and did. But if they could have seen what went on in Reagan's home, the assistance he needed for every little thing, the unrelenting horror for the family, then a truer picture of Alzheimer's for the public would have emerged. Instead of 'how bad can it be?' they'd realize with icy dread what this mysterious and largely hidden scourge 'can be.' If I went public, maybe we could show a truer picture of what Alzheimer's really is--it's not just memory loss. Society has to prepare. I felt like I was screaming from the palisades, yelling at the people playing on the beach, building sand castles, and I couldn't get them to look up and see the tsunami rising on the horizon.

I knew that Maureen Reagan had been given Bernie's tape; and that the President had been shot in the torso. Maybe, because of surgical procedures, he had a damaged omentum, or none at all, plus he may have been too old. I could have been wrong, but it was my speculation that if these things were true, he wouldn't be a good candidate for the surgery anyway, and I certainly had no way of knowing what his family felt--we all make our own private decisions.

February 2000

"Reversing Alzheimer's"

Drew titled the interview "Reversing Alzheimer's" (*) and when it aired in the Greater Los Angeles area, things really hit the fan. Phone calls and emails to me never stopped. Harry was getting hundreds of calls, determined to answer them all. So was the University of Nevada School of Medicine where he holds a professorship, and so was Drew at CBS. The two of them also got a lot of flack from those incensed that they had dared to tell people about such things, giving people false hope. I also heard that medical ethicists were announcing that the surgery was immoral and illegal. If that's their opinion, then they are obviously in the wrong line of work. The ghost of Semmelweiss was still very much alive and well.

For the most part, I was happy with the program. My only negative thought was that it made Bernie look more self-sufficient than he really was, but they did emphasize it was NOT a cure--and that was important to stress.

There were so many requests from the public to see the program that CBS ran it several more times. It was bought by a few other markets--Miami, Seattle, San Francisco--I'm not sure where--and people picked it up on satellite dishes. A friend in a major city told me that she'd called her local station to see when it would air and was told that their medical consultant, a well-know radio medical commentator, said it was an old scam, there's nothing to it, and they would not show it--exactly what the doctor's letter about Bernie to the Alzheimer's Association said was happening. Surprisingly though, they did air it a couple weeks later. Each time it ran, there'd be another flurry of phone calls--and doctors on television telling people to beware, it hadn't been scientifically proven--all the same-o, same-o.

As part of the program, CBS went to the Alzheimer's Association in Chicago for an interview. Knowing that they had received a detailed letter about Bernie and the surgery's success only weeks before, I expected that they'd have something positive to say about the surgery's obvious possibilities. Instead they said that people had to be careful because they couldn't see all the details of this controversial procedure and it was not a place for immediate cure. They went on that it cannot be the answer for the millions of people with Alzheimer's, you can't do four million surgical interventions, and even if it did work, it has only limited opportunity.

I'm sure that the Alzheimer's Association is concerned about all the victims of this dread disease, that is their *raison d'être*, after all, but no one has claimed omentum transposition is an immediate cure--I wish that were so, but it's not. And all four million victims wouldn't even qualify for the surgery any more than all cancer or heart patients qualify and benefit without risk from surgeries that help those conditions. But if omentum transposition helps some people have a better quality of life for a while, then it's wrong to be dismissed so cavalierly. Of course, there were medications--although none could yet match this procedure--but I hoped the Association would be more open minded. Until something better came along, lives were at stake, lives that could be eased.

After the show, the comments I heard the most were that so many people fell for Bernie.

"I just love that man."

"He's so cute."

Well, yeah, and at certain times, they'd be welcome to him.

The full interview ran for thirteen minutes. (*) If you can hear me up there, Mr. Warhol, somebody still owes me two more minutes.

Denial Is More Than Just Another River

Anxious to see what people had to say about the program, I went to the Alzheimer's message boards. *Augggggggh!* Obviously any tree stump with a keyboard can drivel their way into cyberspace, and boy, did they tumble out of the woodpile for this!

In so many words, most people were *not* going to buy it. Even with the before and after videos they saw of Bernie, they were perfectly comfortable in their denial of the obvious. This is the sort of thing, verbatim, that they posted:

Is that the same Dr. Goldsmith pushing his tired old theories again?

She's just a desperate old woman grabbing at straws.

Obviously the man never had Alzheimer's. He was just severely depressed and now that he's getting all this attention after surgery, he's coming out of it.

It's just the placebo effect.

He had Lewy Body Dementia, not Alzheimer's.

So how do they do this? Does the patient sit on a chair holding his own head while the doctor attaches the omentum to it?

No, they stretch it to his head and then play him like a violin.

I've researched this for the past 2 days and there's nothing to it.

Goldsmith has never done any animal experiments or had any papers published.

I'm a doctor and if there was anything to this, I'd have had it done for my loved one. Just stay away from it.

Doctor, I'm so glad you said that, otherwise I was going to consider it for my husband.

If there was anything to it, I'd have heard about it.

One detractor was particularly tenacious. For days I kept answering his negative comments until I grew tired of it and wrote, "*I appreciate your challenge to me, it gave me an opportunity to clearly explain the surgery and its benefits to others on this board. As you know, there is a great divide between caregivers and many doctors. Now I think it's time for us to go on to other things.*"

But he continued. "*What do you mean by great divide?*"

Enough was enough, I didn't answer back. Days later when I again logged on, there were several postings that began: *Let me tell you what she means by 'great divide.'* And did they ever! Of course I knew people all over the world were reading our exchanges, Debby even read them in France, so I was gratified when some wrote in to agree with me. But I never leapt into that particular stewpot again.

One researcher posted that it cannot be a scam. Dr. Goldsmith was not promoting the surgery, no one was promising any wondrous cure, there was no elixir being offered for sale, no advertising for patients--just a statement of a procedure that had been done. He got pilloried, too, poor man. Nonetheless, I know most people are opposed to it, and that's OK with me. I wouldn't encourage anyone to have a wart removed, muchless major surgery. People do what they want to do--always have, always will.

I also posted that I did not appreciate the unkind things being said about us, and assured everyone that my husband's head was still firmly in place where it has always been. Didn't it occur to anyone that I might be sitting at a screen reading their adolescent ignorant dribble? These were fellow caregivers on the boards, some professionals. More than anyone, they knew the horrors I'd gone through with this vicious disease, how could they say such evil things? *We* were not amused.

What annoyed me the most is that none of the detractors called or emailed me to ask about Bernie's condition, to see his medical reports before the surgery, or inquire about what meds he may have been on. No, it was all unsupported comments about a man they'd never met. How could someone dare to diagnose a patient from a TV program, to second guess the dozen or more doctors who had seen him over the years from first diagnosis to surgery?

They seemed to think I'd just read about something, jumped into doing it, and that Dr. Goldsmith bamboozled me. They didn't know that *I* sought out the doctor, not the other way around. How could they know that I knew Bernie's cerebral blood flow was restricted? Did they know the hours--no, years--I sat at this computer researching for *something--anything--*and rejecting everything else I came across? Did they even consider that I *knew* what I was looking for, and that I recognized it when I saw it? Did anyone know that I'd had him in an oxygen chamber? No, they didn't know anything about me, not one of them knew what they were jabbering about--which is really dangerous--and that's the bottom line on that. But I was certainly getting a clearer picture now of how all that baloney went down about Dr. Goldsmith and spinal cord injuries. It just proves that no good deed goes unpunished--but as I've said, my husband has Alzheimer's--so I just brushed their comments off as so many flyspecks--annoying but of no consequence.

Although I continued to lurk and read the message boards, I rarely posted anything, and *never* about the surgery. I was in no mood to start any more go-arounds. I was, however, thoroughly sick of Alzheimer's, sick of living with it, sick of talking about it, sick of reading about it, sick of looking for answers, sick of explaining, sick of research, sick of doctors, sick of writing about it.

And I didn't like the position it had placed me in. Forget the TV appearance and the accolades; *just give me back my life*. But who was I challenging? There wasn't anyone or anything that could give me back my life, but at least no one should deliberately stand in the way of possibly helping others.

Yes, I was desperate--every Alzheimer's caregiver is, but desperate didn't mean that I took leave of my senses--and yes, I grabbed at a straw, but when I read about omentum transposition, I knew which straw I was grabbing for. After all, if a straw can break a camel's back, why can't it save a life? I'd have had to be crazy to let that chance go by.

The Mystery Memo

Shortly after the interview aired, my fax machine printed out this internal memo from the Alzheimer's Association. I never knew for certain who sent it or how they got my fax number.

To: Chapter Communications, Executive Directors... (and others)

Sent: Friday, February 04, 2000, 10:15AM
Subject: Research Update: Omental Transposition

Research Update

TO: Chapter Executive Directors and/or Staff
FROM: Media Relations
DATE: February 4, 2000
SUBJECT: Omental Transposition

We recommend you share this information with:
**Helpline workers*
**Chapter staff who use research information*
**Chapter Board members*
**Chapter Medical and Scientific Advisory Board Members*
This research update is meant to provide you with background and talking points on a procedure called omental transposition that is used to treat Alzheimer's disease on an experimental basis.

WHAT IS OMENTAL TRANSPOSITION?

Omental transposition is complex neurosurgery that involves separating the omentum - a fatty substance from inside the abdomen cavity. During this surgical procedure, a long piece of omentum is threaded through the chest and neck to an opening in the skull. The omentum is then laid directly upon the brain.

The precise mechanism of action is not yet known. A few theories include:

**The procedure increases the blood supply to the brain. Some believe that Alzheimer's disease results from an underlying vascular problem; therefore, increasing blood supply may decrease symptoms of the disease.*

**Omentum secretes enough neurotrophic factors - a family of substances that promote growth and regeneration of neurons - to have a benefit for people with Alzheimer's disease.*

Harry Goldsmith, M.D., at the University of Nevada School of Medicine, Reno, Nevada, is one of the researchers studying this procedure.

NEWSWORTHINESS:

On February 6 and 7, the CBS affiliate in Los Angeles, Calif., will broadcast a report about omental transposition. At this time, we are not aware of any other news organizations interested in this story.

However, we have developed talking points for you to use if the media, donors or other constituents call you about this procedure. We do not encourage you to proactively contact your local media.

TALKING POINTS:

**Use of omental transposition is relatively new for the treatment of Alzheimer's disease. It is complex neurosurgery in which the risks and benefits have not yet been established.*

**At this time, omental transposition is an unproven technique for the treatment of Alzheimer's disease and* *we're waiting for further developments.*

**Because of its complex nature, omental transposition will not be considered widely as a treatment option. However, it may prove beneficial for research observation purposes.*

**Currently, this type of surgery is available only in a few centers.*

Obviously, someone wanted me to see this memo. I had no idea why or how they had a copy of it, but I found it very interesting reading. It was now clear that when I phoned the Alzheimer's Association after seeing the magazine article in November 1998, and they told me I'd have to find the doctor on my own, they knew exactly who and where he was and all about the surgery, including the theory that it may benefit people with Alzheimer's disease because of the secretion of neurotrophic factors, and that increased blood supply may decrease symptoms of the disease, not to mention the possible regeneration of neurons.

I didn't understand why they were waiting for further developments when they wouldn't tell anyone about it and wouldn't support or fund the necessary research--which they certainly should have been doing all along. If they recognized that 'the precise mechanism of action is not yet known,' didn't they have an obligation to try to find out the "how and why"? No, it wasn't a cure, but something was there that could possibly relieve a great deal of suffering. I'm sure they had good reasons, but I was baffled and angry because I would have had it done two years earlier, before Bernie was so advanced, and I'm certain I wouldn't have been alone in my decision.

I was also wondering about the 'few centers' where this surgery was available. Why not share those locations? I had no idea where they were.

Another Side Of UCLA

Dr. Goldsmith had been invited to speak at UCLA. They called and asked me to bring Bernie in for a cognitive test before he spoke. It was arranged that while a dozen or so doctors were meeting in a room, I would bring Bernie in so they could see him and then I'd be asked to leave so they could have their doctors-only discussion about it. That was OK with me. Bernie didn't have to hear everything that had been done to him, and while I'd never have the medical expertise they had, I did smile to myself because I'd had more personal experience with it than any of them.

A few days later I got another call giving me a new room number because they had to move to a larger location. Within days a third call came that it was being moved again to an auditorium later in the day. This pleased me because it showed a lot of interest in the topic and people could come after work.

The night of the presentation the test for Bernie took longer than anticipated and we came into the auditorium as Dr. Goldsmith's slide talk was winding down. We didn't know anyone there except Drew and Larry Greene, (*) the producer and cameraman from the show they did about us on TV. They were filming Harry and we sat behind them.

Harry was answering questions, but when he didn't know the details of one about Bernie's memory, he looked around and said, "If Mrs. Weiss is here, maybe she can answer that for you." I stood up and went to the lectern. There were things I wanted to say and being able to directly address all of these people in the field was a surprise opportunity that I didn't want to let go by.

A mini-mental test is often used by doctors to track a patient's progress. This is when they ask who the president is, what day it is and to count backwards. It is scored on a 1 to 30-point scale, 30 being normal and declining numbers indicating the degree of dementia. I explained that as a wife and caregiver, I had different concerns than medical professionals did. I was more interested in his sleeping through the night, not shadowing me, not screaming at me about other men, having bowel control, not falling, not taking off all of his clothes--things that cannot be measured on a mini-mental scale. These were the sort of things that the surgery had given us, and while I missed his memory and felt sadness about that loss, it was not the most important element in our lives. I could live with memory loss, I just couldn't live with sleep deprivation.

Then someone asked about scars and I said, "Would you like to see my husband?"

Before anyone could respond, Bernie stood up and said, "Here I am." I wanted to gather him up and smother him in hugs and kisses. He'd been taking it all in, now responding in just the right way--a little gasp and stir came from the audience.

Forming A Coalition

Immediately after it was over, crowds formed around us. Off to my left I could see Harry surrounded by people asking him questions. Off to the right, others were talking to Bernie who was eating it up. I wondered what they thought because I knew he really couldn't speak that clearly, but they might just as well see him as he really was, I didn't want anyone to think he was cured. It was all very heady.

Someone was going to establish and finance an omentum research foundation, and a producer wanted to do a movie about us. Everything and everyone that night excited me. It was really going to happen I thought, it was really going to happen. I was meeting people--people who believed and who would help, Harry was getting recognition, UCLA was interested, and my love was so happy--he deserved every bit of all the positive attention.

A Bumble Bee

Bernie and I were still plugging along, and sometimes if he moved any slower, he'd turn into a pillar of salt. It could drive me nuts. "Move," I was always telling him, "hurry up, move faster." And in reply, I swear he'd slow down.

Then there was the day that we walked out of the house toward the car when he suddenly stopped short and warned, "Watch out, there's a bumble bee!" And sure enough, there was one lone monster of a black bumblebee buzzing around his head. He began to swat at it and I yelled, "Hurry, hurry, get in the car!"

Now Bernie *never, never* hurried to get into the car. Often as not he'd open 'Sophie's backseat door, walk in the wrong direction, anything but get in the passenger side--except this time. You should have seen him haul a-- around the car, open the door, jump in, and pull it shut. I think he had his seatbelt buckled before I even got my door open. So you see, lots of time I think he knew darn well what he was doing.

•TWENTY-NINE•

July 2000

After the UCLA talk, things began happening, people pushing for the surgery to be done here, mostly without any input from me. From time to time Harry would call, or someone else I didn't know, just to give me an update on the progress or lack of it.

And then there was a strange phone call from a man who said he showed Bernie's tape to a university professor who is his wife's doctor. He called to console me because the doctor told him that 'the man died.' I had to assure him that Bernie was very much alive. Who starts these rumors and why? Well, a premature death has been reported about countless others from Mark Twain to the Beatles, so Bernie's in good company.

Then I heard that the medical establishment, whomever that may be, was saying that Bernie was "slipping." I can't imagine who that could have been, no doctors had seen him that I didn't know about--who was saying that and why? Wouldn't you think that someone would ask to see him? We weren't hiding. Wouldn't you think that they would be encouraging instead--wouldn't you?

A community hospital in another county south of Los Angeles was interested in doing the surgery. Not that that meant a walk in the park, far from it. All the questions, personalities, meetings, explanations, writings, annoyances, setbacks, and more would have to be done all over again. But things were moving in the right direction.

If all of this came to pass, it was my hope that the story would be given to Drew. But at the moment, it had to be kept quiet. If it got out, the attacks would start all over again, so I felt--and so did everyone else--that it should be kept out of the media, at least until several patients had been done and enough time had passed to report, hopefully, some positive results. It wouldn't be long before so many people knew about it that keeping it quiet would be a good trick. It was my true feeling that there are people out to stop omentum transposition in any way possible and disparage whatever we've tried to do.

My biggest problem, other than anxiety about getting it done, was still the same--it was the people who contacted me all the time wanting to know how to get to Germany, where the doctor was operating, how much the surgery costs, all of it. And I had to tell them the surgery was not being done currently and I could not say if, when and where it would ever be done. More than one person called later to tell me, tearfully, that a mother died, a brother died--and I felt awful that there was nothing I could do. The same thing was happening to Harry, more so, and he couldn't do anything either. No matter where it was done, all the proper channels with their protocols, challenges and changes had to be gone through one by one.

September 2000

When Bernie had his colon surgery, I didn't think the surgeon or the staff listened to me or understood how to handle a patient with dementia, and although everything turned out OK, it still nagged at me. I just don't think you can put an Alzheimer's patient, someone with dementia, in the general hospital population without the staff's knowing that they need special attention, that they cannot respond and react the way others normally do. You can't believe what they say or trust them to do what you want or expect.

When I talked to Debby about this, she thought they could use some veterinarian training because vets are used to caring for and understanding the needs of living, breathing beings in dire straits but who are unable to verbally relay detailed messages about their condition and have no idea what their own vital needs may be. Weird as it sounds, there's a lot to that, but you have to be familiar with the behaviors of Alzheimer's patients to grasp her point.

Current nursing staff at hospitals are certainly familiar with normal patients unable to communicate for the moment, but not familiar with omentum surgery and I'll wager most have never treated an advanced Alzheimer's patient. I hope they will be briefed about what it is, what to expect, and how to treat and respond to their patients--if it finally gets done here.

As an aside, I also worried a lot about the anesthesia on patients with dementia, specifically Alzheimer's, I think there may be a detrimental reaction--at least I believed that to be true from things I'd heard, especially with heart and hip surgeries. Anyway, ready or not, the hospital expected to begin the omentum surgeries by January 2001. It was still all being kept a secret, but the first patient had already been selected.

November 2000

"Reversing Alzheimer's" Follow-Up

Nearly a year after we first appeared on television, Drew did a follow-up program. This time he went to Washington, D.C., to interview the Director of the Alzheimer's Research Centers Program at the National Institute on Aging (NIA) under the National Institutes of Health (NIH). The Director is well known and respected in the Alzheimer's community, particularly his knowledge of gene discoveries and the part they may play in diagnosis--which could be a very critical element in finding the elusive origins of the disease. I also knew he has been at gatherings with doctors who were aware of omentum surgery, so it was surprising that he told Drew he knew little about it--don't these people talk to each other--even if it's only to say negative things about various projects? He said that even if the surgery does work, it probably would get little attention from the NIA, it's terribly expensive, invasive and traumatic, and while it might give some interim 'better quality of life' if it works, it's not the answer to the disease.

I wasn't surprised that he looked ill at ease on camera. I can only speculate on why he said things that didn't compute. By now I knew that few doctors wanted to be publicly involved with any of this, there were careers to consider and, although I could not believe it, I was hearing of promotions denied for those who advocated for it.

If anyone at NIH really knew very little about the surgery, then they weren't doing their job. But of course they knew, all they had to do was take a few minutes to read their own Web site, (http://www.ncbi.nlm.nih.gov/entrez) it's all over the place. As for me, I think that a chance at an 'interim better quality of life' is better than being a vegetable--but, apparently, not everyone feels that way.

He also talked about how expensive it was--well, yes, but if a patient, for any medical condition, needs less care--whether at home or in a care facility--then the cost is going to be *less*. The surgery's benefit then is actually fourfold: (1) in dollars, (2) the well-being of the patient, (3) it's easier for the caregivers, and (4) it's less heart wrenching for the family. Bernie is not on a regime of expensive drugs designed to control bizarre behaviors and mood swings, nor do I take him to a high-priced specialist every few months just to get another prescription, and I no longer pay a king's ransom to a care facility because now I am able to care for him at home.

Remember that before surgery I had Bernie in an assisted living facility paying a base of $43,000 a year, plus extras for helping him shower, groom, have pedicures, and laundry done. The only service I could have possibly done myself was laundry--and that cost was negligible. It was about 40 minutes away and I went out every few days, so the cost of driving and auto maintenance was an added expense. If I had kept him at home it would still cost me about the same. Since he never slept at night--I was beyond exhaustion and no meds made him sleep, and there were no family members who could give up their work and help me on a permanent 24-hour basis--I'd have to hire people for both day and night.

For some time after surgery I did need full time help until Bernie regained his strength. Finally I just had Traci in the mornings at $10,000 a year, and day care at $5,000 a year, so it was costing me $15,000 a year, which was still a lot and I did some fancy juggling to cover it all, but that was instead of $50,000 for a care facility, which my pocketbook thought was a pretty good ratio. I might need more help in the future, I might decide to let Traci go and do what she does myself, or I might decide to work a few hours while Bernie's in day care and bring in money that way--at least now I had options.

So the NIH should understand that I was personally well ahead of the game financially. And if they looked at the government costs in helping to care for such patients, then the government would also be ahead--so we should look at the 'cost benefit ratio' and see the obvious--everyone would benefit!

Just as the Alzheimer's Association plays a major role in doling out research grants in the millions of dollars, so does the government doling out millions of tax dollars, including my contributions. If they each gave a paltry one million dollars, it would pay for itself in no time, there'd be more than enough for clinical trials as well as omentum research. But they have their agendas and their careers. Still, for all the money they toss around, until they come up with something better, it behooves them to help us reach for what they dismisses as 'some interim better quality of life.' Now is that such a bad thing? Well, is it?

A Son Speaks

Also featured on the program (*) was the son of another omentum transposition patient, a math professor in the later stages of Alzheimer's. "You have to understand this," he said speaking of his father, "the word smile was not in our dictionary for five years. He would not know what that meant, he would not smile. The fact is, the procedure works."

To the son, the attitude toward the surgery sounded like a bureaucratic way of saying that Alzheimer's patients and their families were just going to have to wait for something else. He concluded, "If they knew the torture the families and caretakers are going through, they would jump on this. I can't realistically understand what there is stopping them."

Neither can I.

January 2001

"The Best Laid Schemes O' Mice And Men Gang Aft Agley And Leave Us Nought But Grief And Pain For Promised Joy!"

Robert Burns

Although I never saw it, I was told by several people that CBS ran our interview again on New Year's Eve. It was their number one "Special Assignment" report for the year 2000. Drew and Larry (*) won a *Golden Mike* for the show, and later they'd win an *Emmy*. Even though they won awards, and even though it had more viewer response than any other news segment, when Drew went to CBS to try for a national story, he was told there's not enough interest in Alzheimer's--I'm afraid that's the way society still sadly sees it.

It had been a year since we were all at UCLA. Perspective patients and their families were on pins and needles, how much longer could they wait until it was too late? Bernie's symptoms that had reversed themselves were still holding true, though I saw some decline. After all, we always knew he'd still have Alzheimer's, but for the most part, he was doing well at home and in day care, certainly better than he was two years ago.

I realized no one was going to hurry to do any surgery because of me and our being on television. Doctors, and the powers that be, had to have it in their own heads that it might help, they were the experts. Some doctors told me that they knew there was some reversal and they wanted the surgeries done to try to find out how and why--one way or the other. I thought of all those who kept nagging that it hadn't been scientifically proven, it was only anecdotal, so this had to go forward, I could see that, but things were still very much up in the air.

•THIRTY•

"Follow The Money"

'Deep Throat'
"All the President's Men" - 1976

Risk/Benefit Assessment

I had to get a life! I couldn't seem to let it rest, although I had no say, clout, or control over what happened. I felt like I'd been paddling over white water as fast as I could, and every time I saw calm ahead, there'd be an undercurrent that flipped me over. Why did these surgeries for others mean so much to me? Neither Bernie nor I would benefit?

I decided to follow up on something I'd been hearing about--'*risk/benefit*'--find out exactly what that all meant and why I kept being told that omentum transposition did not fit into those parameters. It all tied into Government guidelines used by medical institutions to determine what they will or will not do. This is essentially what I found:

"***Risk:*** *The probability of harm (physical, psychological, social, or economic) occurring as a result of participation in a research study. Both the probability and magnitude of possible harm may vary from mini-*

mal to significant. The federal regulations define only "minimal risk" (see below).

Minimal Risk: *A risk is minimal where the probability and magnitude of harm or discomfort anticipated in the proposed research are not greater, in and of themselves, than those ordinarily encountered in daily life or during the performance of routine physical or psychological examination of tests. {45 CFR 46.102(i)}.*

Benefit: *A valued or desired outcome: an advantage....the risks of participation in research can be expressed as a probability that subjects may be harmed by research procedures while anticipated benefits may express the probability that subjects and society may benefit from research procedures..."*

I also read that these guidelines were not valid under all circumstances; it could be a judgment call. Well, OK, I could understand that, not all procedures have the same value, but I also knew that far more risky research surgeries are performed at hospitals and universities than omentum transposition and, in my layman's interpretation, it would fit nicely within the stated goals.

By way of background, I learned that after any number of medical scandals in the past, the National Research Act of 1974 led to the establishment of Institutional Review Boards (IRB) to monitor all federally funded research projects. In turn, the Department of Health and Human Services created the Office for Human Research Protection to oversee the IRB's. In the decades since, medical research has radically changed and literally exploded. Many IRB's are overloaded with research requests, they can't be experts in every field, members have other interests, and many have their own pet projects that are likely to come up for review in the future. As with everything else, IRB's are easily rife with personalities, conflicts, and politics--maybe judgments sometimes get skewed.

Further, IRB's aside, researchers and scientists need funding, and that money often comes from for-profit corporations, the government, or fund-raising organizations. Not surprisingly, and quite legitimately, these same people often own stock in many corporate companies, and the phenomena of people having financial interests in the outcome of their work also extends to civil servants working in the government, as well as those involved in making decisions about financial distributions from charitable entities, so there can easily be 'conflict of interest.' Too often, conclusions based on what is best for the patient, for the public, isn't always as clear-cut as we have a right to expect. And I question just how much all these layers of agencies established to protect us are really doing such an objective job.

I have never been a conspiracy buff, I believe strongly in coincidence--things just happen--but then there are lobbies, PACS, soft money, donations, mutual backs to scratch, hospitals, research labs, doctor groups, associations, grants, boards, lawyers, drug companies, investors, conferences, agreements, organizations, profits, insurance companies, politics and sometimes--things don't *just* happen.

I can think of several entities with reason to stop omentum transposition--but that's only my speculation--and that of people who have given me their opinions. Anyway, I'm not interested in pursuing that part of the story and have no intention of alluding to or mentioning any specific group because I don't know--I really don't. But it is grist for someone else's book, and if I were to take that route--which I won't--I'd use the following approach as a starting point.

To find the culprit, the French say *cherchez la femme*, but we pragmatic Americans say, "Follow the money."

◆THIRTY-ONE◆

April 2001

(Shanghai, China)

The Chinese Man Who Bites His Wife

The Chinese were starting a ten-patient clinical trial and Harry had gone to Shanghai to operate. The way things were going here, and depending on how they handled any publicity, the Chinese would get there first while we Americans were still puttzing around. Some of the feedback I'd gotten from nay-sayers was that Dr. Goldsmith only operates in Third World countries like China, so anything from there would be dismissed as having scant merit. But I no longer considered China a Third World country, and from all that he personally told me, neither did Dr. Goldsmith.

Harry had spent a lot of time in China, had several long-time colleagues and a couple of Honorary Degrees. The Chinese had been using omentum transposition successfully for spinal cord injuries, and for treating encephalitis and post cerebral anoxia (cerebral palsy) with some good results. *(The Omentum: Application to Brain and Spinal Cord)* (*)

Harry had no say in the choice of Alzheimer's patients and was surprised that those presented for surgery were very advanced, having mini-mental scores of something like 2 or 4 with the highest around 12. Some of them were also of an advanced age, maybe in their 80's. The patients would be checked from time to time to monitor their progress, but while he was still in China, Harry had already noted improvements after surgery in some of them. The most dramatic was a man who spoke absolute gibberish and grabbed his wife and bit her every time she came near. As a caregiver myself, I cannot imagine how impossible it would be to live in such an untenable position. Nonetheless, a few days after surgery the man once again knew who his wife was, he no longer bit her and was speaking clearly.

I teased Harry, "How do you know that he was speaking clearly, you don't understand Chinese?" Well, he clarified, that's what the doctors told him. It pleased me no end to realize that somewhere in China a woman was no longer being bitten by her husband--all because I went public--and she didn't have any idea that I existed!

(May 24, 2002)

Letter From China Forwarded To Dr. Goldsmith And Then On To Me

Dear Prof. W. and Dr. Z.

How are you! B.L., the dementia patient has been developed since last Jun 19th when he underwent the omental transposition to the brain. The most improvement is that he is no longer incontinent. Now I describe the improvement.

1. *The thinking and response is quicker, language is abound with logic-like making jokes with others.*

2. *Can distinguish person and make out persons name.*

3. *More amenable and friendly to greet guest.*

4. *Mood is more stable and is able to sit and lie for more time calmly.*

As he is getting better more and more, the dementia hospital now takes pictures of him as the paradigm of improvement.

I bet you must be happy when know this. Just like the farmer get harvest.

Best regards to the American doctor!

Best Wish.

C.F. (the patients wife)

April 2001

Brian's Opinion

One day I received this email from the pole vaulter Brian Sternberg. Even though he was talking about the surgery for his personal spinal cord injury, I think it belongs here in this book about Alzheimer's. The surgery offers improvement to enough patients to make it viable. It's not a cure, I keep stressing that, no one says it's a cure--but it *can* help--how can anybody ignore giving people a chance at a better life, at some improvement? He wrote:

"...I've seen some of the fine reports of the tremendous advancements made by Bernie. It's AWESOME! Somehow more people have to find out about the tremendous improvement that's available from omentum transposition...

It's amazing how it's helped ME! Just being able to spend as much time as I do at this computer is a good example. The thing I have to be extremely careful of is not sitting up TOO much! I have one of those chairs that tips back, and it's difficult to remember to do that often enough.

Having the omentum surgery done has really helped me in another way, too. Prior to having it done my voice was so weak people had to lean over and put their ear right in front of my mouth to hear me. My voice is nothing great now, but it's FAR better than it was. I can easily join in on a conversation with half a dozen people, and I'm able to take and place telephone calls with a headset 'phone (like telephone operators use).

Keep lookin' up!

Brian"

Causes

If you wanted to make a gazillion dollars, answer, "What causes memory loss, dementia?" Sometimes there's the obvious: head trauma, stroke, depression, meningitis, AIDS, syphilis, alcoholism, amnesia, brain tumors, fluid on the brain, dietary deficiencies, certain medications, metal poisoning, aging, environmental toxins, less oxygen in modern air, a virus--but many are 'iffy' explanations, because sometimes some of them can be reversed. Get on the computer, start researching, drive yourself crazy.

Then there are all the obvious--Alzheimer's, Huntington's, and Parkinson's; or vascular dementia, sometimes called multi-infarct dementia--which just comes on without apparent reason, or might come from a stroke, chronic high blood pressure, cardiovascular disease, or diabetes--none of which Bernie has ever had, unless he possibly did have one or more silent strokes. There are frontal lobe disorders and weird little conditions with weird funny names that hardly anyone has ever heard of: Lewy Body Dementia, Pick's Disease, Wernicke-Korsakoff, Binswagner's, Creutzfeldt-Jacobs Disease, a form of 'mad cow' disease--of all things--and don't forget diminished blood flow.

There's always talk about mercury fillings, aluminum cookware, fluoride, diet, various supplements, vitamins, exposure to chemicals, deodorants, hair dye, sugar substitutes; the need for keeping mentally active, exercise; magic secret discoveries that only cost $$$ a bottle, and on and on, it's everywhere. But, if you believe, as I do, that Alzheimer's has been with the human race for hundreds of years, if not more, then it is unlikely that it is caused by any of these modern-day issues.

To explain Alzheimer's, you have to open your view to include other cultures where people don't have fillings, who use different cookware, and aren't exposed to our chemicals--but they still get Alzheimer's. What's the commonality? And what are the percentages of Alzheimer's in other countries, and do they differ? What about Harry's patients in China who have the same disease Bernie has but a totally different life style? Oh, there is *always* a reason, a cause for everything, of course, but finding it, subduing it, well, that's another story.

Regardless of the cause, when it is unknown--or sometimes even when it is known--the only reasonable thing to do is try to treat the symptoms, keep the patient comfortable and maintain as much calm as possible for everyone in the house--not always the easiest thing to do. The problem, obviously with so many variables, is that what works for one patient is no guarantee it will work for another, so you try this and try that and hope for the best, and the undeniable upshot is that, with Alzheimer's, so far, not all that much helps.

Maybe it's residual from a childhood disease, like getting shingles if you've had chickenpox. We know these things stay in our body. If you can be left sterile or get a heart murmur from a childhood illness, why not something left in the brain? And sometimes I think it's having a 'half-empty glass' personality, being unable to relax and have fun, always anxious, pessimistic--or maybe one is that way because the Alzheimer's is already there.

Well, if I had the money to put on it, I'd go for a recessive gene as the culprit, that's how I think it began with Bernie, the propensity was there and unrelieved stress brought it out. Keep the focus on DNA research, see if it is feasible to finally pull out destructive genes without causing any other damage. Stop it before it begins.

A Good Marriage

Since I have lived in this time warp of Alzheimer's, the rest of the world has continued to move along paying little attention to Bernie and me or to all those others suffering--and it is a dreadful suffering--the ravages of Alzheimer's. Most people don't understand, don't care, and just go on with their own lives. Why not? It's an old man's disease, isn't it? Besides there are all those other equally devastating diseases. Everyone has their sad story. I'd have done the same thing--that's how ignorant I was about Alzheimer's.

I saw all of Bernie's odd behaviors, people told me things, but at the same time, I didn't see it, I didn't listen, it just slipped through my mind. I believed there were valid reasons for everything. Stress, work distractions, male hormones--guys are strange creatures, you know.

I loved him. He was good, decent, protective, loving, smart--we loved each other, had great kids, a good life--we could never hurt each other. But we had a lot of problems, too, and I'll never know how much of it was due to Alzheimer's? Sometimes it was apparent, but most of it was so vague it can hardly be described.

On occasion, determined to break through the wall I thought Bernie had built around himself and get to the bottom of it once and for all, I'd talk to him, ask questions, try to analyze things--I'm very pragmatic. But it was pretty much all one way, he didn't resist, just never seemed to understand my probings. I got angry, thought he was being deliberate, although that was never his nature. It was like digging in a ton of fluffy white feathers, I never got anyplace and when I thought I'd reached the bottom, I just fell right through.

Twice I dragged him to marriage counselors; it lasted no more than two or three sessions. Bernie went straight to his lawyer, telling him they were going to tell me to leave him, and the lawyer agreed, then he came home and told me about it. The weird part is that the counselors did tell me to leave, but I never mentioned it to him or told anyone until now. How did he know that?

'Leave him now while you're still young enough and pretty enough to get another man.' That's what they said, and while I didn't mind being called young and pretty, I thought it was the most stupid advice I'd ever heard. I wasn't interested in 'getting another man.' I wanted the one I had, to save my marriage and my home--not destroy things, and never a murmur from them about the children, the negative impact it would have on them. Their lives would be torn apart, taken from the comfort and security of their home; I'd probably have to work full time, leave them alone a lot or with strangers, leave our house, be exhausted, worried about everything and not have Bernie in our lives, at best a week-end father. No! I wanted to be with him, I wanted us to all be together--I wanted my home, my family, my life--stupid 'experts' didn't know squat. Just dump the life you've built and start all over with another man--as if that would be so easy. They were 'divorce' counselors when I wanted 'marriage' counselors.

But, how would they have known that they might well be dealing with a brain disease, they saw what they saw and no way to change things. And supposing they did know in those early years, when no one thought or talked about Alzheimer's. What if they had said, "I'm sorry, dear, but your husband is exhibiting signs of Alzheimer's, so get out while the getting is good."? I'd have held on tighter than ever, never left, I couldn't abandon him any more than I knew he would never abandon me.

Of course, I'm not saying that all of our misunderstandings or disagreements were due to Alzheimer's, all couples have their marital conflicts and we were no exception, and I was not always the most agreeable mate--but it did add to things, kept me confused--and maybe Bernie as well. There were so many times when he said I didn't tell him something that I thought I had, that I would doubt my own recall. Without realizing it, I was changing, accommodating myself to living with a disease that I didn't even suspect was hiding under the surface of our lives.

And then there were so many puzzled questions people asked me. "Why did Bernie say that?" or "Why did Bernie do that?" It annoyed me, I'd toss off, "Why are you asking me, ask him!" I never knew what they meant or how I was supposed to respond. I never saw anything wrong.

One morning, I think Bernie was about 24, I got a phone call from his foreman at work. It may have been decades ago, but I never forgot it. The man, who I didn't know, was telling me that something was wrong with the way Bernie responded to things. He told me very clearly that I should take him to a doctor! I thought that the man might be setting Bernie up, somehow, trying to make sure he didn't compete for his job--or some such thing! He talked for some time and I just held the phone in astonishment, saying nothing.

Over the years, I've thought about that call many times. What was he trying to tell me, and would I have even believed him? In those days no one knew the word 'Alzheimer's.' I think he knew something was wrong, maybe he'd seen the same signs in someone like his father, he was trying to forewarn me--but of what, he couldn't clearly say, he didn't have today's vocabulary, and I would have had no understanding, anyway.

Supposing I got Bernie to a doctor. I'd say, "His foreman said to bring him in, and 'no' I don't know why." After an exam, the doctor would have said that there was nothing wrong with him. So I did nothing, and looking back, I don't think it made any difference.

And, I never told Bernie. I didn't want to create conflict between the two of them at work.

Forty, fifty years ago--what would you have done?

•THIRTY-TWO•

Tuesday, August 28, 2001

"I May Not Have Gone Where I Intended To Go, But I Think I Have Ended Up Where I Intended To Be"

Douglas Adams

As it happens, the Omentum Research Foundation was established (*), but in spite of my upbeat feelings, UCLA passed on the surgeries and the movie was never made. But outside of the Shanghai study, there had been six omentum transposition surgeries done for Alzheimer's. The first one was done here in the States, the other five were abroad. Five of the six patients showed noticeable improvement, one barely and only briefly. One died 31 months after surgery, another died a couple of months following surgery, both were elderly men and deaths were from unrelated causes. Most patients and their families have chosen to remain anonymous, which is understandable, however, a paper by Dr. Goldsmith describing all six patients before and after omentum transposition was published in *Neurological Research, 2001, Volume 23, September (*).*

This was a special day, though. We finally got our first omentum transposition surgery for Alzheimer's done by Dr. Goldsmith here in the United States since the first patient in 1993. It was done in the county hospital south of Los Angeles, and it didn't take three or four years as I'd originally been advised--it took less than two years since I'd gone public in November 1999. I was told that this is quick for a new procedure, and I take that to reflect at least some doctors have a real interest and belief in realizing something very good can come of this.

The day after surgery I went to see the patient, a middle-aged woman. Harry was there along with some of her family. Although her eyes were closed, she looked terrific, hale and healthy--well bandaged, of course, obviously still drugged from the operation. When told that I was there, she smiled, and when her husband leaned over and told her how beautiful she was, her smile widened. Thankfully, it appeared that she was not going to have all the post-op problems that Bernie had in Germany, and unlike Bernie who had absolutely no memory of his surgery, she was well aware of hers. Whether it was because she wasn't as advanced, or didn't have to endure an arduous flight, or something else, I certainly didn't know, but I was impressed when she was already walking to the bathroom in a couple days.

A couple weeks after her discharge she returned to visit the hospital nurses who had taken care of her. All were suitably astonished at how well she was doing. They, of course, had never seen this surgery, so they didn't know what to expect. Later her husband told me how her behaviors had improved, she was a much calmer person, and no longer needed all the anti-psychotic drugs she'd been taking. No, she wasn't the woman she once was, but in his words, "Just her being less agitated was worth the price of admission."

Now that the dam had been broken, I had hopes that others would do some surgeries as well, that this was only the beginning of good things yet to come. I'd come to learn that in the medical world it all takes time and money as well, but it's hard to be patient when you know that others can be helped *today*.

So there was progress, still in secret--silly to have to hide this way, but it looked like the things I wanted might come to pass--surgery in the States, omentum research, and an established fund to get it all going.

Excerpts From A Letter From The Husband Of A Woman Who Had Omentum Transposition Surgery In The States

Over twenty Alzheimer's patients have had omentum transposition since I went public, about half in the United States, half abroad. Dr. Goldsmith wrote a summary of them, *Treatment of Alzheimer's Disease by Transposition of the Omentum*, (*) published in the November 2002 Edition of the Annals of the New York Academy of Sciences. Personally, I only know a very few of them and nothing about the rest, except that most--not all--but most reversed many symptoms.

Dr. Goldsmith:

Since her operation on 10/30/2001, K. has shown what I feel is tremendous and steady improvement in her ability to function in society. Some of the things that she has regained the ability to do are.

Remember the Day, Month and Year.

Prepare a basic meal without assistance (cook meat, veggie and starch).

Simple shopping.

Travel to the local store alone for one or two items.

Count money.

Cares for grandchildren for short periods of time.

Follow a movie plot.

Reading continues to improve.

Remember familiar places.

I could continue to list the little day-to-day improvements but would sum it up by saying "you have given me back my wife."

K. still gets frustrated from time to time but I feel this is due to her mind outpacing her ability to effectively and quickly communicate. She has just started occupational speech therapy.

We are planning a vacation in the Fall. This would not have been an option if K.'s Alzheimer's continued at the pre-operation rate. We still have a long way to go but there is a light at the end of the tunnel.

K. recovered from the surgery quickly and to my knowledge has suffered no ill effects.

Our family cannot put into words the gratitude we feel for all that has been done for K. and how it improved our quality of life.

Thank you.

C.S.

And From A Wife About Her Husband

Dear Dr. Goldsmith:

October 4, 2001 was a day that changed the immediate future of my husband D. and the rest of our family. From a news report in Los Angeles, our family learned of omental transposition as a possible treatment for Alzheimer's Disease....We all knew....the surgery carried with it many risks. However, facing....the likelihood of an inevitable decline in his condition, he was willing to take that risk.

The surgery was successful, but with his extra thick omentum there was a setback....this was not expected and very upsetting. Working with the excellent surgical team....and outstanding therapists....I am happy to report that D. has shown continuous improvement.

It has been 9 months since the surgery. We as a family, and D. himself, see marvelous changes. We have our husband, father, and friend back in our lives....There is indescribable joy and excitement as he amazes us with his new achievements....He can tell you who the mail is from. He picks out his own CD's and engages in thoughtful conversations. He's begun speaking in longer sentences....He is more frustrated at the things he still can not do, but we feel this is a tremendous progress. As before the surgery he did not see his decline. While all these physical improvements are a thrill for us to see come back, nothing is more fantastic, more thrilling than the return of his personality. The return of D! As he has said many times since the operation, "I am coming back."

We are all very thankful for this privilege given to us, and hope the outcome of our effort will help others in the future as it has helped us.

Best regards,

S.M. and children

Reading these letters I think that both patients improved more than Bernie and certainly did not have the same post-operative trauma as he had in Germany. I don't understand how anybody can read these letters without getting goosebumps, how those who actively discredit the procedure can sleep with a clear conscious when they know, absolutely, that it can relieve so much suffering--even if it's not for everyone and not a cure.

The Argument

In the over fifty years Bernie and I have been together, we've had many difficult disagreements, but our usual arguments were for us to simply give each other a wide berth, to keep our distance and our mouths shut until things blew over. So I was very surprised one day when he got frustrated and angry while I was helping him get dressed. It had happened before, but this time my resentment and self pity had been building all day and I turned angry in return, called him names and let him have it. "You're impossible," I snarled. "I don't have to do this you know, I can just leave and let you take care of yourself, then you'll see all that I do for you, I'm just going to leave." I turned and stormed out of the room, fuming. He followed me down the hall, taunting, "Go ahead, leave, get out of here!" Most of the time he had trouble stringing too many words together, but he clearly got those suggestions out!

His response brought me up short and left me laughing to myself. After all these years, it took this misbegotten disease for us to actually threaten each other with leaving--we'd never done that before. And, once again, it told me that he was still in there, still aware of what was going on between us, and he wasn't about to let me get the best of him.

◆THIRTY-THREE◆

September 2001

Nearly three years after surgery in Germany.

"In Three Words I Can Sum Up Everything I've Learned About Life: It Goes On"

Robert Frost

Since I hadn't been visiting Royale as often, I really hadn't seen how much Bernie had deteriorated before the surgery, and the condition of each patient before surgery would have bearing on the outcome. But three years ago Bernie was confined to a mental institution and drugged into a stupor--anything was better than that.

All of his improvements were a surprise to me because I knew he still had Alzheimer's, that he'd likely continue to decline. I understood that dead cells could not be reanimated, and I doubted anyone really knew what dormant damage had already been done. I wanted to know the progress of those surgery patients who were not so advanced, to see if their decline would be pushed further away and the improvements extended for a longer period. And I especially hoped for real progress on the research project. Although, in fact, while I believed things were happening, I never asked anyone and didn't hear very much about any of it. I did learn for certain, though, that programs were started, doctors ready, patients examined and then someone would come put the *kabash* on everything and, no, I can't imagine why anyone would dash the hopes of so many desperate people when there was a chance they could be helped.

Bernie got better, a lot better, then about two years after surgery there began a decline that continued up and down. Mostly he was OK, but sometimes he could simply be out of it, his eyes wouldn't focus, and he was completely confused about everything, but most of the time he was right there--that's the nature of the disease. I knew there were people who thought they'd rather be dead than live the way that he did, and in the past Bernie may have felt that way, too, but not since the surgery. I knew Bernie and I knew that with all the fears, frustrations and sadness he'd had, he'd still rather be alive, he wouldn't prefer to be dead, not for a minute. The truth is, we were doing just fine.

Sometimes he looked at me from behind the face of a bewildered little boy. I could almost hear him say, "Mommy, I'm afraid. I don't want to cry, but tell me, I don't understand." And I didn't understand either. An explanation would be nice, but I didn't have one. Instead he got what I could give--protection, security, love and affection--to the best of my ability. And while I saw the confusion and fear, he never indicated that he wanted out--he was still brave, accepting his lot, coping, willing to go on--and I was willing and wanting to go on with him.

He had a decent life, not the one that he'd had before Alzheimer's, but it was a nice little life, certainly better than many people have. He was usually content, even happy. He lived in his own home with his wife and dog who greeted him with a bone at the back door on the afternoons when he came home from 'work' so he could give her a joyful scratch. He was well cared for, clean and warm, slept safely, enjoyed his food, going to day care and being with people who loved him. These were substantial blessings.

If I Had To Choose

For a while after surgery Bernie did very well on standard cognitive tests and while I understood their overall importance, they had scant impact on our daily lives. It didn't matter to me if Bernie could recall past presidents. At home, such mental tricks were so far removed from our daily reality that they didn't even cast a shadow of a blip.

If I had to choose between his counting backwards or sleeping through the night, I'd choose sleeping; if I had to choose between how many animals he could name in one minute or not shadowing, I'd choose not shadowing; if I had to choose between his knowing what day it was or not raging at me about being unfaithful, I'd choose his not raging. I knew that many of these behaviors eventually passed, anyway, as the disease progressed in some patients, but most of these changed shortly after surgery and happily they were still holding. They weren't something that could be measured on any sort of cognitive scale.

Sleep: *This was the worst thing for me, his keeping me up all night and at me all day, being sleep-deprived. Now he had a normal sleep pattern. Times varied, but he usually went to bed around 8:00 p.m., and woke up around 6:00 a.m.*

Raging: *He never stopped raging and threatening me before about being with other men, yelling about* *divorce and my being unfaithful. He never did that anymore.*

Constant repeating: *He didn't do that anymore.*

Paranoia: *This was common, 'they' were in the house, but that was gone.*

Falling: *He fell frequently and hard. Royale was always calling to tell me they were taking him to the doctor because they thought he needed stitches or broke something. Now he never fell.*

Violence: *Before surgery he was so violent he was a danger to others and had to be sedated into a stupor. It took some months for the violence to finally subside after surgery, but he never needed anything more than half a Xanax to quiet him down in 15 minutes or so. Now he only got agitated on rare occasions and that was almost exclusively in the shower, if he was confused about my helping him dress, or had a rare bowel mishap. He could get wild-eyed, grab my wrists and say vile things--mentally he just left the realm. But within minutes, as soon as the shirt was on, the shower over, he'd be as calm as ever. It was just a matter of his not always understanding what someone was trying to do for him, his fear and frustration, so I'd agree with whatever he said, promise him anything, speak soothingly and finish the task as quickly as possible. If he was particularly difficult, I just walked away and he soon calmed down. It was better to leave everything on hold for a few minutes and not escalate his frustration by insisting something be done immediately.*

Sundowning and Shadowing: *He did both all the time, now he didn't do either.*

Undressing: *He used to take off every stitch of clothing and walk around stark naked. He stayed properly dressed all day now.*

Imaginary mites and shadows: *He used to 'pick' them up all the time, but he didn't do that anymore.*

Dozing: *Frequently dozed or slept. Now he'd take a morning nap after breakfast, but otherwise stayed awake all day.*

'Sophie': *Wouldn't respond to his dog at all. Now he treated her normally, and was pleased when she greeted him at the back door after his return from day care.*

Stooping: *He used to walk with a prominent stoop and very slow, feet shuffling, arms hanging loose. Now the stoop is usually gone, the feet and arms move normally, but he again walks slowly.*

Senses: *For a couple of years his visual perceptions appeared to have returned to normal, but they were getting bad and that had a negative impact on many things he did. He could still read signs and seemed to understand them, but that was about it. Sometimes he would not make eye contact, but other times he was bright eyed and alert. He usually responded to loud and unexpected noises, but not to someone's voice, didn't always turn toward them when called, had trouble understanding what he'd been asked to do and getting his limbs to respond. Sometimes his skin seemed much less sensitive to temperature changes and wetness. Since he ate well and turned away food he didn't like, I assumed his sense of taste and smell were normal.*

Speech: *At first, much of his speech came back, but never returned to normal. His voice was stronger though, but it was an effort for him to articulate clearly,* *he couldn't get out the right words. Strangely, if he was half asleep or angry about something, his speech was usually more definite. Still, he often got out the correct words in a short sentence, just couldn't carry on for very long. He knew that and compensated by making silly joking sounds.*

Grooming: *For a long time he was able to shave, brush his teeth and dress himself. But then he didn't always know what a toothbrush was for or how to use it, the same with his shaver. His sensitive skin made it harder to keep him clean-shaven. He'd fuss if I tried to shave him, but, thankfully, he'd let our son do it. Sometimes he resisted in the shower, but he usually washed and dried himself and seemed to enjoy it. Because he couldn't always control his movements, dressing him could be a challenge, but he was mostly cooperative, and again, if he was angry, he'd put his clothes on easier by himself.*

Socializing: *He continued to go to adult day care and eagerly greeted the driver when the van came to pick him up, he knew the people there, enjoyed the socializing, and also knew family and friends. At a holiday dinner in our home, he was just fine, no one would suspect there was anything wrong with him.*

Incontinence: *He lacked bladder control, but usually had some bowel control. For a while after surgery, he was able to take care of himself, but then he couldn't find the bathroom and dealing with his clothes confused him. However, I could tell by the time of day and his behavior when he needed to use the bathroom. Thankfully, bowel mishaps were rare and it was never like it was at Royale where he messed in the hallways and smeared stuff on the walls.*

Eating: *His appetite was good. Even though he drank daily food supplements, he stayed thinner than* *ever, but he was still strong and healthy. Usually he ate by himself, but sometimes he'd be in the middle of a meal and I'd help him finish; unless it was ice cream or other sweets, then he always cleaned the plate.*

All in all: *Obviously there had been a decline over these almost three years. He was not as alert, didn't always know where he was, what he was expected to do, and had slowed physically, but then he was getting older and had been through a lot. And while I knew that he understood much more than he could express, he was not always 'there.' Still, the difficult behaviors that made it impossible for me to care for him at home before surgery were all gone now.*

It was hard to assess just where Bernie was. I knew that some of his behaviors were the usual symptoms of late-stage Alzheimer's, and yet, he was still functioning pretty well and so far had avoided the anguished tortures that plague so many others. I was often asked, "How often do you have to take him to the doctor?" Basically, I never took him, but maybe once a year to his psychiatrist so she could, in her words, 'eyeball' him.

But there was one funny incident. She wanted to get a brain scan to see what changes there'd been since he'd had the first one years ago. I was waiting in the reception room when the doctor reading the scan came out and asked, "What did you do to that man?" No one thought to tell them before the scan about the surgery, and they had no idea what they saw in his brain--the other end of his omentum!

Three years ago the doctor in lockdown told me he could live another ten years. One never knows, of course, but for however long he was going to be here, it was clear on balance that the improvements from surgery far outweighed any negatives.

Doesn't Aricept Do The Same Thing?

Aricept, and other meds, are very beneficial for many patients and that's wonderful. But Bernie was sedated into a stupor in a locked down mental institution. He was rapidly sliding into the final abyss, and no doctor ever mentioned giving him Aricept once he passed the early stages.

Omentum transposition reversed the most severe symptoms of the disease in its latter stages. In addition to bringing a laundry list of biochemicals and adult stem cells to the brain, the surgery will also allow drugs to breach the blood brain barrier and possibly make them more effective. Some argue that overriding this natural protection is theoretically dangerous, but the patient is going to die with Alzheimer's anyway--at least give him a chance for a little better life in whatever time is left. Current drugs don't appear to be able to produce these dramatic outcomes on their own, maybe something soon will, but in the meantime, we have the ability to relieve a lot of suffering and it behooves the medical community to do so.

Someone claiming to be a doctor once posted on a message board that he'd like to see a trial where half the people get Aricept and half have omentum surgery to see how each group fared--he was betting there'd be no difference. I answered that I thought that was a fine idea. Set it up, fund it and you'll have plenty of volunteers. It didn't surprise me when there was no response.

Bernie Has An Adventure

Bernie was in a car accident with a friend, fortunately no one was hurt. By the time I reached the scene, everyone was assembled at a nearby gas station--police cars, tow truck, ambulance, flashing lights, all the people, and I could see Bernie milling around with the rest of them. He was obviously OK, thank goodness, and seemed to understand all that was going on. He wasn't frightened or upset. When all the information had been exchanged and everyone was getting into their vehicles to leave, Bernie turned to me and said clearly and definitely, "I'm going with *you.*" I was just so pleased and proud that, without my being there, he handled all the excitement and strange people so well.

January 2002

Los Angeles, California

"And Will You Be Happy, Charlotte?" "Oh, Jerry, Don't Let's Ask For The Moon, We Have The Stars"

Bette Davis & Paul Henreid
"Now, Voyager" - 1942

It was Sunday, the one day I was alone with Bernie, and every Sunday, by 8:00 a.m., I was ready to take him to the nearest care facility, leave him there and never look back. I had to prepare his breakfast, and I would rather stay in bed; I had to get him dressed, and I would prefer to sit in my robe at the kitchen table with my coffee and argue with the newspaper. 'Sophie' would be sitting next to her empty bowl with a woeful expression, so I had to take care of her, too--and I just wanted to be left alone!

But I sighed and played the martyr--as if I had a choice. Finally, after everyone had eaten their *petit dejeuner* and Bernie was settled in for his morning nap, I phoned Debby in France. She was doing French to English translations for some of Jean-François' maps, Guillaume would graduate high school by summer and Justin was buying snowshoes. I offered to send him some old tennis rackets to use instead, but he declined my generosity.

Later, I piled Bernie and 'Sophie' into my ancient Pontiac for a drive along the coast to watch the winter waves frost the shoreline, then a brief tour around the duck lagoon where 'Sophie' cast the birds a bemused eye from the back window, and finally, a stop at the drive-through for burgers and fries.

At home, I divided the food among the three of us and we ate watching some sport or other on TV until Matt and Zeli came by. While Matt shaved him, I could hear Bernie laugh in the bathroom and before they left he got some happy bear hugs from Zeli.

Night comes early in January. Once in bed, Bernie asked me if I was coming, too. So I slipped off my shoes and curled up next to him still fully clothed. "This is nice," he smiled, then as he fell asleep, barely managed, "I love you." And I forget all about a care facility--at least until next Sunday.

Not every day was so idyllic, not by a long shot, but overall, I'd have to say it had all been worth it because Bernie and I are not some flickering romantic voyagers on a movie screen, we're just ordinary real people who live, breathe, laugh, love, cry and hurt. Like millions of others who have also been grievously assaulted, we can never rise again whole to play out another role. For now, we must anchor here, albeit in this relatively safe harbor. And although our personal voyage isn't over just because these pages close, I know this absolute--Alzheimer's is hard, it's very hard, harder than most people realize. But there are worse things in life--far too many worse things that hurt far too many people--so for now, I won't ask for the moon, I'll settle for the stars.

♦AFTERWORD♦

February 2002

Los Angeles, California

Traci had left before Christmas for a family emergency in Belize and didn't come back. Once again I was doing it all alone. I was forced to face our future one more time. I thought about the problems of getting another part-time caregiver--and there are always problems. Not all are reliable, much less truly caring. But more than that, I was simply running out of steam, even the thought of trying to hire someone was an effort I didn't have the energy to make. It was going on ten years and I was aging, not really able to care for myself as well as I should--everything was always Bernie and his needs first.

Although he was certainly better than before surgery, it finally became too much for me, even if I got help, and I knew it would not get better. Inside my skin, I could feel my whole body shaking. I thought it would only be a matter of time until I began to shake outside as well, to stumble over words, fall into caregiver dementia--it happens--do something really stupid, and I was having stress-related medical problems. I knew that I needed respite to get myself back together. A few weeks should do it and there was a very fine care facility less then ten minutes from home.

Bernie was very happy in this new place, never asked about going home, participated in a few activities, became friends with some of the patients and staff. Often I took him out for a meal or an ice cream sundae. Sometimes it was just a ride, and if I brought him to our house, he seemed indifferent to it. Now he always recognized the facility as I brought him back, got out of the car sprightly and went straight inside.

It was working out better than I could have imagined. In fact, on Valentine's Day the following year, he was elected by the staff as their favorite male patient. He was given a cape, a crown, and a bag of candy which he promptly ate. He took off the crown but wore the cape all day. He gloried in all the special attention. He not only had awareness of what was going on in the facility, but he was always happy to see me and his other visitors. He wasn't on any meds and I believe none of this relative ease would have been possible before the surgery.

I had hoped that the surgery would be readily available in the States to help others, but it hasn't worked out that way, and frankly, I don't have the energy or the need to fight the good fight any more. Let the medical establishment fuss or not about it. This book is meant to tell people about the impact of Alzheimer's, to have a record of what happens to an ordinary family struck by such a difficult disease; the surgery, while important, is really just a peripheral part.

In time, I began to feel the constant strain leaving me and, finally, with a sense of profound sadness and great relief, I let him stay at the facility for the foreseeable future. He was only minutes away, well cared for, popular and quite happy.

July 27, 2003

Although there was some slowing down, things went along pretty well for over a year. Then more and more I'd find him dozing on a couch when I'd visit. He'd wake up well enough to share some treat I'd brought, smile and respond, we'd walk around the facility, go for a ride, but the decline was there. I found it harder and harder to rouse him to walk, so I'd sit with him, share the goodies, let him sleep, hold his hand, rest my head on his shoulder and tell him over and over how much I loved him, how important he was, and he was always so pleased in return. One afternoon he perked up briefly, smiled at me and clearly said, "You're beautiful." I understood that he knew exactly who I was. He never spoke again.

I wasn't feeling much concern, it had all become our normal way of life. He seemed to have dropped to another plateau but was still eating by himself in the dining room, responding, so I was a bit surprised the day I found him dressed, but resting on his bed, seeming a bit more tired than usual. Still, he got off the bed to sit in a chair while I fed him his lunch. He ate almost all of it. A chest x-ray has been ordered and came back negative. So I wasn't worried.

The next day, Bernie was again in bed, laying on his side, with a nasal tube for oxygen. Now I had some concern, although his breathing wasn't all that bad, just from time to time a bit rapid. I curled up in his back in our familiar spoon-fashion, my arm holding him close. He was calm and quiet, breathing all but normally, sleeping comfortably. I felt his chest breathing, his body warmth, took in his smell and held him closer.

Debby was supposed to come for a visit from France in three days. I needed to find out what was happening, no one had volunteered any information. And when I asked the nurse, she was evasive, not giving me a direct answer. Finally I insisted that she tell me his true prognosis--I wanted to know if Debby would be here in time. I insisted and insisted, wouldn't leave her side until she told me, "I don't think he'll last three days."

Well, I didn't believe that at all, he didn't seem weaker. That's not what I wanted to hear, what my eyes told me. Lunch came, we took off the oxygen tube when he pulled at it and he ate with relish. He responded to the differences between meat and cake, drank without a problem, and was breathing perfectly fine. Although he had a blank stare, he knew I was there. After a while he went back to sleep and I left, confident that he'd be OK for now.

The next morning I came back to see that he ate breakfast. The nasal tube was gone and now he had on an oxygen mask, but his breathing still didn't seem to be laboring. The nurse said he was failing. I kissed him, straightened his hair and ran out to the desk to call Matt. When I returned in only a minute, the nurse said, "I'm so sorry, Betty." I didn't understand, he still had the oxygen mask on, and then his arm fell lifelessly from across his chest. It was over but I continued to kiss him.

The staff finished their tasks and asked if there was anything they could do. I knew there were things that must be done, but I told them 'no,' and so they left us alone. There was no hurry. Sitting against him on the side of his bed I put his arm across my lap and, knowing it would forever be the last time, I began to stroke it, feeling the familiar soft roughness of the hair on his forearm, as I'd done so many countless times before. For a precious moment, I was alone with him to silently cry. Soon Matt and Zeli would arrive.

"A Dying Man Needs To Die, As A Sleepy Man Needs To Sleep, And There Comes A Time When It Is Wrong, As Well As Useless, To Resist"

Steward Alsop

People ask me how Bernie died, was it peaceful, in his sleep, did he know, was it painful? I don't know if he knew, I think not--I prefer to think not. He appeared to me to be sleeping, 'out of it.' I have no way of knowing how much awareness he had, what he may have been thinking or feeling, he never opened his eyes, I never heard any sounds. There was no gasping for air, thrashing about--I don't have to know what it feels like to stop breathing.

That was always the plan, there was never going to be any prolonged suffering if it could be avoided. The decision had been made years ago when Bernie and I were young, healthy, confident and completely in the dark about what life had in store for us. The DNR order was always in place. At any time, I could have rescinded it, but things moved so quickly I honestly didn't think about it. There just wasn't anything to do--no pneumonia to treat, no infection, no heart attack--he just stopped breathing.

Yes, he could have been taken to the hospital and put on a breathing machine, he might have lived that way for a few more days or weeks, but it would not have been peaceful then, not for him, not for us. If he had awareness, he'd be frightened and confused, we'd all be full of anguish and despair. Considering what I'd seen of other Alzheimer's patients in the care facilities, of what I've read on Alzheimer's computer boards, I think we were blessed that Bernie went as he did. And he never got as bad as he was before the surgery, I was grateful for that.

We'd long ago said our good-bye's as I lost him over and over, so many times in so many ways in so many years--and I know he knew that, too. He knew he was leaving. And I'm certain about one more thing, nothing was going to restore dead brain cells, he'd never be any better. Nature made the call and I chose not to interfere. Nature was kind--his death was peaceful, not painful, frightening or prolonged. He deserved that peace and dignity.

A Final Sacrifice

Bernie had been through too much to just let everything be buried with him and so I called UCLA to get a brain biopsy performed, to see if anything could be learned from the omentum surgery. Dr. Goldsmith came from Nevada to supervise and the procedure was done by their chief of neuropathology instead of the usual technician. Brain tissue samples were sent out and will be studied here and abroad by those interested in trying to find out how and why it worked. I realize it is far from the final answer, but somebody is bound to learn something from it.

And, not incidentally, his Death Certificate gives the Cause of Death as "Alzheimer's."

Dr. Goldsmith continues to operate, mostly in Berlin, Germany where they are more than pleased to have him do the surgeries that America's medical establishment tries to stop. He has performed 22 omentum transposition surgeries for Alzheimer's since Bernie's; 6 showed no improvement, 16 did improve and of those, 8 improved significantly, as Bernie did, and all are still doing well. Many patients were well advanced, so any improvement is remarkable. Those are very good odds--16 out of 22, and I'd do it again for Bernie in a minute--only wishing it would have been done sooner before so many precious cells were lost. It is also critical to mention that none of the other patients were slow in waking up and responding normally after the surgery--just Bernie--but it was only a matter of days and then he was fine.

Today there is much talk about embryonic stem cells, and sadly, it has become politicized. It is a medical, moral and ethical situation, it should not be political. Everyone has a right to their opinion without being pilloried by those who disagree.

Our stem cells do not disappear, we carry them with us forever and adult stem cells are found in many parts of our own bodies including the omentum. There are also stem cells in umbilical cords. And while there is research going on with adult stem cells, it gets little publicity. From my layman's point of view, I think that it's a better option.

Bernie lived for four-and-a-half years after the surgery, three of them in his own home with me where he had a lot of good times and frequent contact with so many others who also loved him. He would not have lived that long without the surgery; and I know it contributed to his gentle death and the absence of so many of the more common and tragic symptoms of advanced Alzheimer's. I'll be eternally grateful for those few precious years--as I know he was, he enjoyed them immensely.

The rapid loss of dying brain cells was stanched, at least enough to make a significant difference. If you attempt to diminish one part of the brain's function, it's likely to affect the other parts as well, and so I believe that any meds used in trying to control his violence would have done him in sooner.

Matt talked about his father's final sacrifice at his funeral, how the biopsy may help others, and we all knew that's what he'd have wanted. Bernie always fixed things, and if he could help fix the brain, he'd feel really good about that--that's pretty important, and not such a bad legacy.

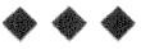

MEDICATIONS PRESCRIBED OR RECOMMENDED FOR BERNIE

From the first diagnosis in August 1993 until his death in July 2003, these are medications either prescribed or recommended for Bernie. Some of them he never took, others were discontinued almost immediately. Few seemed to help for any length of time, most made his symptoms worse.

Aleve
Alprazolam
Aricept
Aspirin
Ativan
Chelation
Cognex
Depakote
DMSO
Folic Acid
Ginko Biloba
Haldol
Lorazepam
Melatonin
Neurontin
Papaverine
Paxil
Propranolol
Prozac
Remeron
Risperdal
Testosterone
Trental
Vitamins C & E
Xanax
Yohimbine
Zoloft
Zyprexa
& countless supplements

HARRY SAWYER GOLDSMITH, M.D.

P.O. Box 493
Glenbrook , Nevada 89413 USA
Phone: 775-749- 5801
Fax: 775-749--5861
hlgldsmith@aol.com

CURRICULUM VITAE

EDUCATION:

1952	Dartmouth College, A.B. Hanover, New Hampshire
1956	Boston University School of Medicine, M.D. Boston, Massachusetts
1956-57	Intern, Surgical Service, Boston City Hospital, Boston, Massachusetts
1957-58	Junior Assistant Resident, Surgical Service, Boston City Hospital
1958-59	Senior Assistant Resident, Surgical Service, Boston City Hospital
1959-60	Senior Resident, Surgical Service, Boston City Hospital
1960-61	Chief Resident, Surgical Service, Boston City Hospital

FELLOWSHIPS:

1959-60	Research Fellow, Department of Anesthesia, Boston City Hospital
1964-65	Research Fellow, Sloan-Kettering Institute for Cancer Research, New York

POST GRADUATE:

1963-65	Senior Surgical Resident, Memorial Hospital for Cancer & Allied Diseases, New York

LICENSURE;

New York	#009015E
Pennsylvania	#011707E
Delaware	#888
New Hampshire	#2716
Massachusetts	#25082
California	#55348

CERTIFICATION:

1961	American Board of Surgery

MILITARY SERVICE:

1961-63 Captain, U.S. Army Medical Corps
1961-62 Chief of Surgery, Seoul Military Hospital, Korea
1962-63 Staff Surgeon, Fort Devens, Ayer, Massachusetts

SOCITIES & ORGANIZATIONS:

American College of Surgeons
A.O. Whipple Surgical Society
James Ewing Society
International Society for Study of Esophageal Diseases
Society of the Sigma XI
Society for Surgery of the Alimentary Tract
New England Surgical Society
Central Surgical Association
International Melanoma Group (Sponsored by World Health Organization)
British Association of Surgical Oncology (Pancreas Club)
Societe Internationale de Chirurgie
Society for Vascular Surgery

ACADEMIC:

1958-60 Assistant in Anatomy, Boston University Center, Boston
1960-61 Senior Teaching Fellow in Surgery, Boston University Medical Center, Boston
1961-62 Instructor of Surgery, Soodo Medical School, Korea
1964-65 Assistant in Surgery, Cornell Medical School, New York
1965-67 Instructor in Surgery, Cornell Medical School
1968-70 Director, Surgical Education, Memorial Hospital for Cancer & Allied Diseases
1967-70 Assistant Professor of Surgery, Cornell Medical School
1970-77 Samuel D. Gross, Professor & Chair, Department of Surgery, Jefferson Medical College, Philadelphia, Pennsylvania
1977 Distinguished Professor of Surgery, Jefferson Medical College
1977-83 Professor of Surgery, Dartmouth Medical School, Hanover, New Hampshire
1983-95 Professor of Surgery & Adjunct Professor of Neurosurgery, Boston University School of Medicine

RESEARCH:

1966-67 Assistant Director of Surgical Research, Memorial Sloan-Kettering Cancer Center, New York
1965-68 Assistant Clinician, Sloan-Kettering Institute for Cancer Research
1968-70 Associate Director of Surgical Research, Memorial Sloan-Kettering Cancer Center
1970-77 Director of Surgical Research, Jefferson Medical College

CLINICAL:

1965-66	Clinical Assistant Surgeon, Memorial Hospital for Cancer & Allied Diseases
1966-68	Assistant Attending Surgeon, Memorial Hospital for Cancer & Allied Diseases
1968-70	Chief, Gastric & Mixed Tumor Services, Memorial Hospital for Cancer & Allied Diseases
1968-70	Assistant Attending Surgeon, Memorial Sloan-Kettering Cancer Center
1970-77	Surgeon-in-Chief, Thomas Jefferson University Hospital, Philadelphia, Pennsylvania
1970-87	Consultant Surgeon, Memorial Sloan-Kettering Cancer Center
1977-83	Attending Surgeon, Mary Hitchcock Memorial Hospital, Hanover, New Hampshire
1983-95	Boston University Medical Center, The University Hospital, Boston
1996-present	Clinical Professor of Surgery, University of Nevada School of Medicine, Reno, Nevada

OTHER POSITIONS;

1976-88	Editor, Goldsmith's Practice of Surgery (12 Volumes), Harper & Row, Lippincott, Publishers
1988	Honorary Degree, Shanghai Second Medical University, Shanghai, China
1990	Editor, The Omentum - Research & Clinical Applications Publisher - Springer-Verlag, New York and Heidelberg
1995	Honorary Degree, Xuzhou Medical College, Xuzhou, China
2000	Editor, The Omentum - Application to Brain & Spinal Cord, Publisher - Forefront, Wilton, Connecticut

Dr. Goldsmith has published 225 papers and contributed many chapters to medical textbooks, especially pertaining to the omentum.

He spent many years performing omentum research on animals before applying it to humans.

WARNING SIGNS OF ALZHEIMER'S DISEASE

(http://www.alz.org)

Alzheimer's would be simple if it was only a matter of being forgetful--everyone forgets something sometimes--especially in a society as complex as ours. Unfortunately, the early signs of Alzheimer's are not easily recognized or taken seriously, even by doctors. It's expected that some people get a little pixilated as they age--it's no big deal.

But sometimes it *is* a big deal--a very big deal, and the family that takes a loved one, *old or not so old*, to a physician at the first vague signs is well advised. It may be something else that can be reversed or controlled and it's good to find that out right away; but if it is Alzheimer's, then it's vitally important to get the patient on medications as soon as possible and develop a plan of care and action as the illness continues to develop. If you feel your concerns are being dismissed by the doctor, get a second opinion--don't let it go, find out what the problem is.

1. Memory loss: On occasion, almost everyone will forget an appointment, names and phone numbers but will eventually remember later; the Alzheimer's patient will not remember later nor even remember that he forgot.

2. Difficulty performing familiar tasks: Things that were always done automatically will become impossible. Making a simple sandwich is too confusing; how many slices of bread, what to put on them--do you use a fork or a spoon, where does the lettuce go, does the tomato slice go on top, how do you get the meat inside? People with Alzheimer's will be unable to operate household appliances safely or participate in lifelong hobbies.

3. Problems with language: From time to time, we all forget words but they'll often come back in the middle of the night; Alzheimer's patients not only forget words for simple objects, they will often substitute another word that may be close but incorrect. A 'car' can become a 'bus' - a 'fork' will be called a 'dish' – the 'lawn' may be a 'rose' – a 'toothbrush' will be 'that thing for my mouth.'

4. Disorientation to time and place: It's normal to forget the day of the week, especially around holidays or maybe forget where you're driving, but those with Alzheimer's can get lost on their own street, even in their own house when they can't find the bathroom. They don't know how they got someplace and have no idea how to get back home.

5. Poor or decreased judgment: No one always has perfect judgment but Alzheimer's patients dress without regard to the weather, wear two or three shirts, set out for work with pants over their pajamas or wear underwear on top of their street clothes. They easily lose money or give away large amounts to someone on television, a telemarketer, or paying bills they don't owe.

6. Problems with abstract thinking: Numbers become very confusing; they cannot remember the value of what a number represents. Alzheimer's patients won't be able to make change, figure out a receipt, how to leave a tip or balance a check book.

7. Misplacing things: We all lose our car key, forget where we put that very important paper so it'd be easy to find, but eventually we usually find most things. But it is especially difficult with Alzheimer's patients who often 'hide' things--that you may never find--and then they accuse others of stealing their things. Or they put a shoe in the microwave, the scissors in the refrigerator.

8. Changes in mood or behavior: Everyone has occasion to feel sad or moody, but those with Alzheimer's can swing rapidly from happiness to tears or calm to anger--and often for no apparent reason.

9. Changes in personality: Sometimes, as people age, they may get a little sweeter or nastier, but with Alzheimer's people not only get confused, they become suspicious and fearful. The most lifelong independent person can turn very dependent, usually on only one particular person.

10. Loss of initiative: On occasion everyone gets bored and tired of the same routine--housekeeping, work, social events--same people, same things, same activity, but with Alzheimer's the patient may become very passive, seemingly unable or unwilling to do any of the normal activities, just sitting in front of the television--not really watching or involved in what's showing--or sleeping the time away.

A CHECK-LIST OF WHERE TO START IF A LOVED ONE IS ACTING STRANGE AND YOU SUSPECT ALZHEIMER'S OR ANOTHER FORM OF DEMENTIA, OR IF SOMEONE TELLS YOU OF THEIR CONCERNED OBSERVATIONS AND SUSPICIOUS

Although most families find it all but impossible to speak of such things, if your loved one can still make rational decisions, it is wise to discuss how he wants the problems handled that will arise when he can no longer make financial and medical choices. You might want to consider taping these conversations in the event someone challenges your decisions.

___ If you don't already have them, get Power of Attorney for both financial matters and health care. The problems of your loved one's being unable to handle finances and make reasoned medical decisions for himself will arise sooner than you think. Someone has to have access to finances in order to pay for medical and long-term care when needed. Although you can get forms at office supply stores or on-line, an elder law attorney can be very useful. An attorney can also advise you about guardianship, wills, government issues and other such matters.

___ If your loved one is taking any medications, make arrangements for you or someone else to see, in person, that the right meds are being taken at the right time, that they are not being missed or doubled up because your loved one forgets--and, no, a phone call is not sufficient, you cannot rely on what someone with dementia tells you on the phone to be accurate. The same with special pill dispensers, they only confuse patients who will tell you they are taking their meds, but likely, they are not doing it correctly.

___ Start researching local, state, federal, private and volunteer programs to get as much assistance as possible. Find and visit some adult day care centers, talk to the staff there, this is often a wonderful source of comfort for both your loved one and yourself. Contact your County's Department of Aging for assistance.

___ Look into a variety of residential care facilities in case you need to use them in the future. Try to find one that suits your situation but remember that few places can provide the full-time attention you give your loved one. However, as time goes on, visits with your loved one should become more enjoyable and less stressful if you are not always exhausted from being on call 24/7.

___ Develop a friendly relationship with the doctors--but don't hesitate to speak up, get a second opinion or find other doctors if you are not happy with the ones you have. Many doctors are woefully under equipped to handle patients with dementia. Because of new privacy medical regulations, make arrangements to be sure you are able to talk to the doctor about your loved one. Many of them, rightfully, are uneasy about patient privacy. Go with your loved one to the doctor, hopefully, into the exam room. Your loved one won't be able to give the doctor accurate information and will forget what he is told before he walks out the door.

___ If you are not the primary caregiver, make sure that whoever is gets a lot of support and respite, try to keep the caregiver from burnout or illness, and if it's you--take care of yourself first--and, no, that will not always be easy. Try not to fuss and waste precious energy with family members, it's not always easy with so much added stress, but now's the time to stick together and help each other if at all possible.

___ Seek out support groups and counseling for both you and your loved one. If nothing else, get onto an on-line support group. Type 'Alzheimer's message boards' into your computer's 'search.'

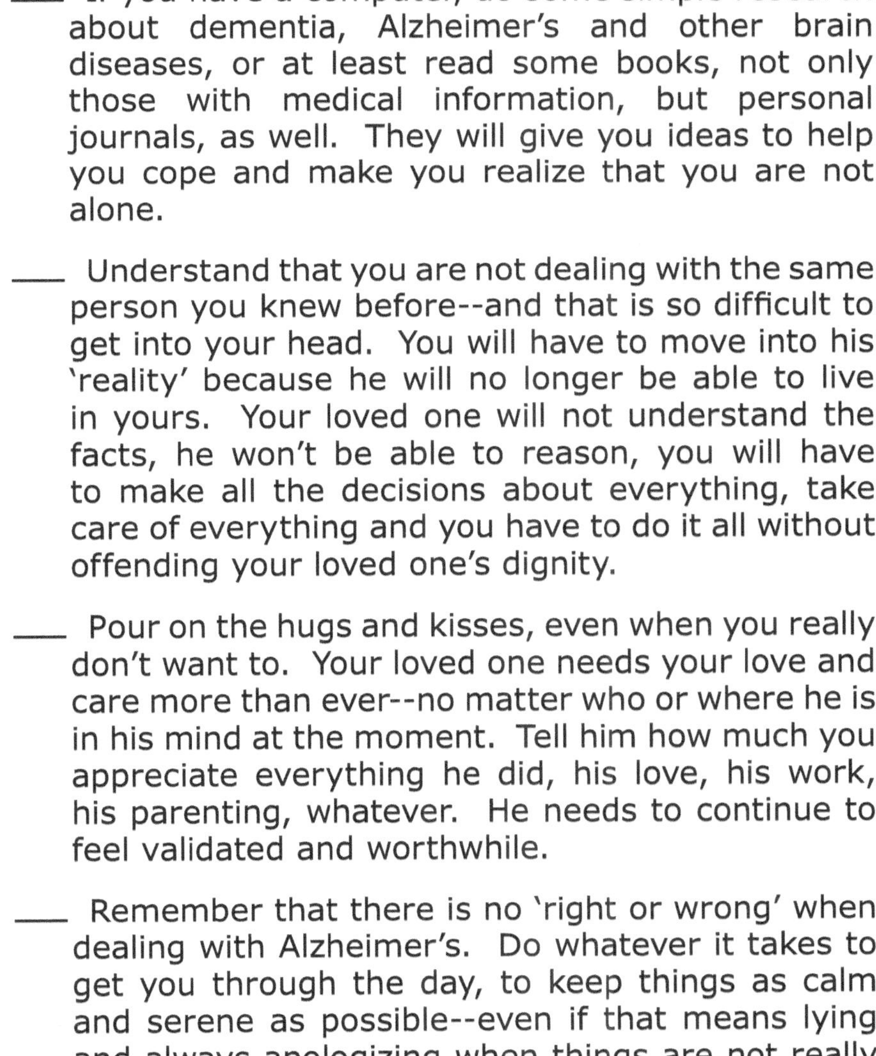

___ If you have a computer, do some simple research about dementia, Alzheimer's and other brain diseases, or at least read some books, not only those with medical information, but personal journals, as well. They will give you ideas to help you cope and make you realize that you are not alone.

___ Understand that you are not dealing with the same person you knew before--and that is so difficult to get into your head. You will have to move into his 'reality' because he will no longer be able to live in yours. Your loved one will not understand the facts, he won't be able to reason, you will have to make all the decisions about everything, take care of everything and you have to do it all without offending your loved one's dignity.

___ Pour on the hugs and kisses, even when you really don't want to. Your loved one needs your love and care more than ever--no matter who or where he is in his mind at the moment. Tell him how much you appreciate everything he did, his love, his work, his parenting, whatever. He needs to continue to feel validated and worthwhile.

___ Remember that there is no 'right or wrong' when dealing with Alzheimer's. Do whatever it takes to get you through the day, to keep things as calm and serene as possible--even if that means lying and always apologizing when things are not really your fault.

FINDING REFERENCES

**"Decreased Senile Plaque Density in Alzheimer Neocortex Adjacent to an Omental Transposition"* (pg. 157) published in *'Neurological Research' - copies* can be requested from:

Norman R. Relkin, MD, PhD
Department of Neurology and Neurosciences
Weill Medical College of Cornell University
New York Presbyterian Hospital
428 East 72nd Street, Suite 500
New York NY 10021, USA

**"Comment on Omental Transposition for Alzheimer's Disease"* (pg. 158) published in *'Neurological Research' - copies* can be requested from:

J. C. de la Torre, MD, PhD
Department of Neurosciences
University of California, San Diego
9500 Gilman Drive
La Jolla CA 92093, USA

*Videos of the television interview "Reversing Alzheimer's" with Drew Griffin (pg. 288) can be requested from:

CBS Special Assignment Producer
Phone: 1-323-460-3131

*Tragically, on September 6, 2002, while on assignment in the Persian Gulf, Larry Greene (pg. 297) was killed in a Navy helicopter accident.

*Omentum Research Foundation (pg. 322)
P.O. Box 92389
Pasadena CA 91109-2389
Email: omentumresearchfdn@earthlink.net

Request reprints of:*

"Neurological Research, 2001, Volume 23, September" (pg. 322) and

"Treatment of Alzheimer's Disease by Transposition of the Omentum" (pg. 324) from:

Harry S. Goldsmith, MD
University of Nevada School of Medicine - Reno
PO Box 493, Glenbrook, NV 89413, USA
Phone: 775-749-5801 -- FAX: 775-749-5861

**The Omentum - Application to Brain and Spinal Cord"* (pg. 312) (Chapters 11 & 12)
Harry S. Goldsmith, MD - Forefront Publishing

ALZHEIMER'S: AN INTIMATE PORTRAIT

and

WHEN THE DOCTOR SAYS, "ALZHEIMER'S"

http://geocities.com/caregiving4alz

ABOUT THE AUTHOR

Betty Weiss continues to live in her same Los Angeles home along with young men from a nearby university who rent rooms and keep things busy and lively. Matt, Zeli and Estella recently moved down the block from her with their doggies, 'Indy' and 'Lola.'

Debby and Jean-François remain in the Pyrenees with Guillaume, who is at a university taking engineering courses, having the same innate mechanical qualities of his Big Daddy; and Justin, a dedicated skate-and-snow boarder, just starting his university life to study urban planning; and 'Nueve' the cat.

'Sophie' still rockets through the house, while out in the yard sweet red tomatoes ripen on the vine and little hatchlings are being born.

www.ingramcontent.com/pod-product-compliance
Lightning Source LLC
Chambersburg PA
CBHW030002190526
45157CB00014B/85

* 9 7 8 1 4 2 0 8 5 7 9 5 5 *